12.99

top to toe

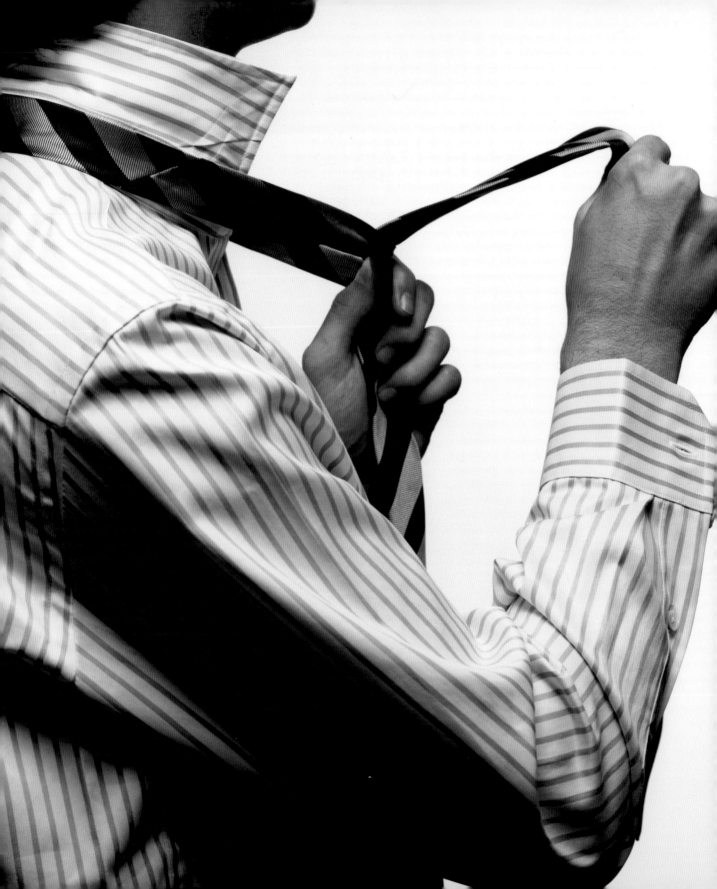

top to toe

The Modern Man's Guide to Grooming

Tony Glenville

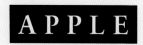

First published in the UK in 2007 by
Apple Press
Sheridan House
114 Western Road
Hove
East Sussex BN3 1DD
www.apple-press.com

ISBN 978 1 84543 191 4

This book was conceived, designed, and produced by
IVY PRESS LIMITED
The Old Candlemakers
West Street
Lewes, East Sussex
BN7 2NZ, UK
www.ivy-group.co.uk

Creative Director Peter Bridgewater
Publisher Jason Hook
Editorial Director Caroline Earle
Art Director Sarah Howerd
Senior Project Editor Emily Gibson
Designer Simon Goggin
Photographer Calvey Taylor-Haw
Illustrators Anna Andrews and Wayne Blades
Picture Researcher Shelley Noronha

Printed and bound in China.

1 3 5 7 9 10 8 6 4 2

CONTENTS

INTRODUCTION

The Valet or Gentleman's Gentleman

In the past, a valet would spend a great deal of time on the maintenance of a gentleman's wardrobe: folding, brushing, and checking clothing for imperfections, sending and receiving laundry, and so forth. Another task was laying out the correct clothing for occasions that might involve several changes during the day. Finally, a valet would offer advice on etiquette, dress, and other such details of the gentleman's day that might otherwise lead to unwise decisions in behavior or apparel. Today it is rare to have full-time staff to perform such operations and, indeed, our lives do not demand such excess of sartorial splendor. Nevertheless, what to buy, what to wear, when to wear it, how to wear it, and how to care for it, is for many men still a conundrum. With the absence of a valet to whisper in your ear or perhaps give a wise shake of the head at an inappropriate decision, this volume offers a view of the gentleman's wardrobe of today, from a valet's perspective.

Right: Checking the details will always be an important part of good grooming.

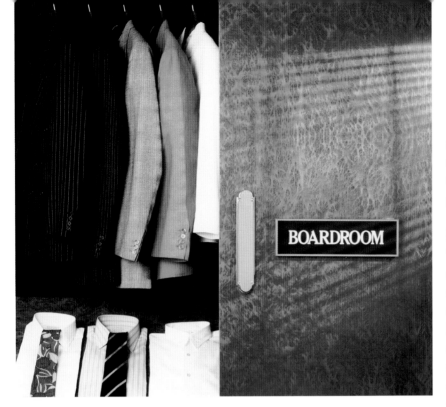

Unless you are a true fashion victim (that is, a man who buys the latest fad, wears the most extreme version of each new style, and lacks individual taste and style, merely following what designers throw in front of him) menswear is relatively circumscribed in its elements. The city, casual, country, and holiday wardrobes contain many of the same items; it is the color, fabric, and details that change. This limited and edited wardrobe has at times led to revolution: the radical 60s, dress-down Fridays, and so on; but in the final analysis, it is the rules that make the gentleman's wardrobe successful. The man who works within their framework will be both confident and at ease in a variety of situations.

Above: An untidy wardrobe, like an untidy desk, will never support a successful career.

MAINTENANCE OF THE GENTLEMAN'S WARDROBE

There is no point at all in spending time and effort on grooming yourself if the clothes you put on are soiled, crumpled, or inappropriate. After spending time and money on a well-balanced, versatile wardrobe, it behooves you to look after it. Throughout this volume you'll find suggestions on storage and maintenance to make your purchases last longer and to insure that you are as well-groomed as possible, even on a limited budget.

THE RULES OF THE GAME

Many situations within both business and leisure are out of the ordinary: gala nights at the opera, fundraising charity barbecues, or special sporting events are not day-to-day occurrences. Since you are unlikely to have a valet to check for you, the best advice is to check for yourself. A swift phone call or e-mail may save you from a potentially embarrassing faux pas. Discretion is truly the greater part of valor when it comes to gentlemen's attire.

FASHION AND STYLE

"Style remains while fashion changes" may sound a little simplistic, but it is true that cutting-edge fashion and an over-fondness for being absolutely of the moment can lead to an inappropriate outfit. By being overdressed or simply too challenging in the attitude you project through your clothing, you run the danger of alienating people, especially in business. Even within the fashion business, too heavy a reliance on being the first to wear a style can label you as a fashion victim, trying too hard, and simply being a slave to fashion with no personal style. So on the following pages fashion is allied with style rather than being a goal within itself.

A FINAL WORD

Further reading and advice will support your learning, but you must be prepared to work at your personal style statement. Trying on clothes, shopping, and reading style magazines may not be your cup of tea; however, if you do so, the results can pay dividends, not only in confidence and the impression you create on others, but also in your professional life. It is surprising how much attention is paid to the style package you present to both your colleagues and your superiors in the workplace.

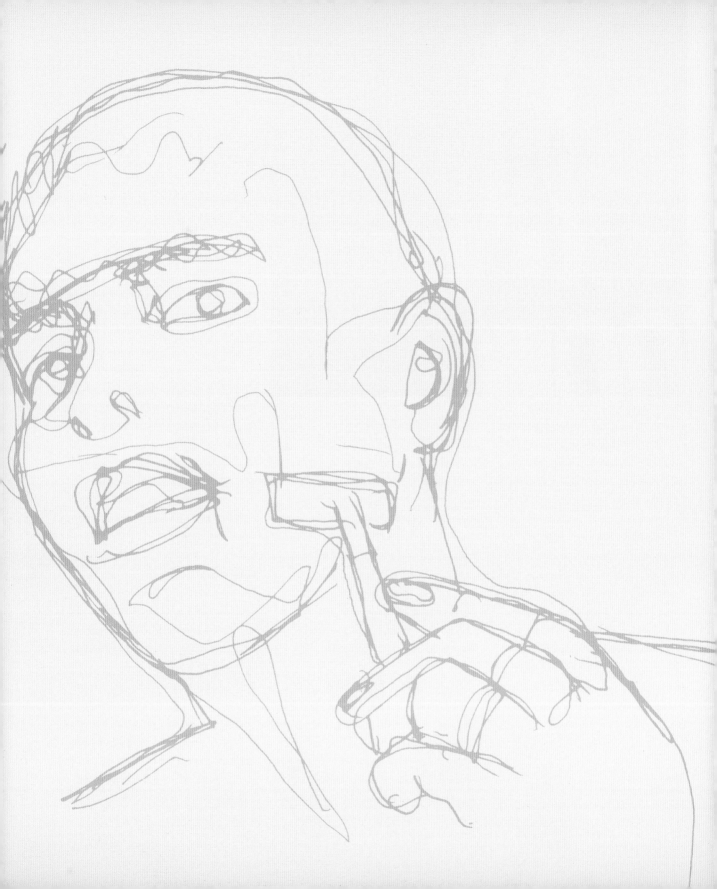

"I admit it was difficult to get men interested in personal freshness, fragrance and skincare products, but the market is growing, as men have come to understand that smelling good and having skin that's comfortable and pliable is not effeminate but smart."

ESTÉE LAUDER, FOUNDER OF THE ESTÉE LAUDER COSMETICS COMPANY

THE FACE

Reactions to your looks and personality start with the presentation of your skin, eyes, mouth, and also your hair, which forms the frame for your face. The individual elements that make up your face may not be outstanding; but if they are sufficiently well looked after, the overall impression can create a sum that is greater than its parts. Both professionally and personally, pride in your appearance, and especially your skin, is not vanity, but a sign that you wish to make the best impression, both for yourself and for those around you.

SKINCARE The skin on your face is exposed to a variety of challenges. These vary from hot and cold through wet and dry to natural and artificial. Climate variations, environmental shifts, and lighting all affect both the texture of the skin and its appearance. Historically this mattered very little to the majority of men. It was not considered "masculine," by common definition, to worry about the effects of working on a farm or at sea, out in all kinds of weather and exposed to the elements at their roughest; nor to consider the damage done to a man's skin in a heavily populated and polluted city. This belief has changed and is continuing to change, although not for everyone. The shift to skincare for men is still in progress and there will continue to be new developments, of which you should keep informed by reading and observation.

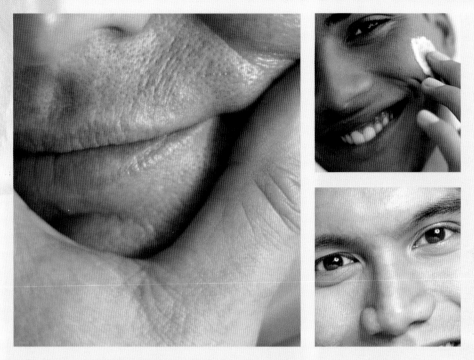

Above: Regular soap can irritate your face, so it is imperative that you always use a specialized skin cleanser, and follow up with a moisturizer. Keep in mind that individual areas of the face may require special treatment: sensitive skin around the eyes, blackheads around the nose, or dry skin close to the hairline.

FACIALS AND TREATMENTS Ever since the earliest days of the gentleman barber, hot towels, facial applications, and treatments have been available. Today there are literally thousands of options and places to go for skin treatments, so make sure you select an establishment with good credentials and some years of experience. There they will be able to analyze your skin and recommend the correct treatments, which may often take place over a period of time. Remember that your lifestyle and especially your diet will have a strong effect on your skin and you must be honest with anyone trying to help and improve your skin.

EYES The skin on different areas of your face has very different qualities of texture and elasticity. The area around your eyes is the most sensitive and delicate area; the texture reflects tiredness, diet, and the day-to-day experiences of your life more quickly than any other skin area. Eye gel and cream specially formulated for this area are now widely available. Some of these products are specifically targeted at men and are well worth investigating.

Tip *Always consult a professional skin specialist for continuing problems that require expert advice to cure and correct.*

NECK Men can suffer from aging and sagging skin in the neck area. There are new preparations that have been successfully developed to counterbalance loose or textured skin in this area. If this is a particular problem area for you, be aware that you can also achieve a firmer appearance through exercise, to keep the underlying muscles toned.

Tip *Extreme procedures, such as peels and cosmetic surgery, should only be undertaken if you have complete confidence in the reputation and skill of the practitioner.*

SHAVING

For many men, shaving is a ritual that is carried out automatically day after day. Often one of the first actions of the working day, shaving may be done in a semi-comatose state at an unreasonably early hour. Yet the importance of shaving well and caring for the skin during the process cannot be too heavily emphasized. A badly shaved face sporting sections of beard missed by the razor, dry flaking skin, and a generally uncared-for appearance are a disaster for any gentleman.

STUBBLE The unshaven look is popular with many men for a variety of reasons: making a rugged statement, accentuating the facial contours, creating a change of look from workday grooming, or simply giving the skin a rest from shaving. Stubble still requires some attention, though; it should be spotlessly clean and free from dryness. The outlines often need attention to give a groomed but casual look, which may include shaving the neck only or simply using an electric shaver to tidy the surface of the stubble area.

Tip Always shave using a mirror that is well lit and that allows close examination of the face during the procedure.

ELECTRIC RAZORS AND BEARD TRIMMERS Some men prefer to use electric razors exclusively, or just for a second shave of the day before going out in the evening directly from the office. Goatees, beards, and sideburns can be kept neat with electric trimmers. After use of any of these appliances, some form of moisturizer or skin balm is recommended. Always keep razors and clippers spotlessly clean and well cared for; it is best to replace them at regular intervals. Do not wait until they start to develop operating problems.

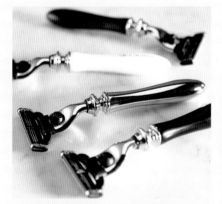

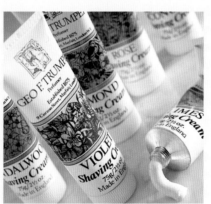

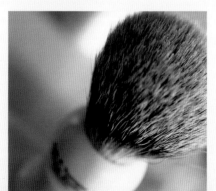

Above and left: It is worth taking time and trouble when composing your shaving kit. Buy good quality razors and change the blades as soon as they begin to dull. Use shaving cream recommended for your skin type, and always use a shaving brush: the bristles will make the hairs stand up, giving you a closer shave and helping avoid shaving bumps. You may pay for rushed or unwise purchases with a shaving rash or inflammation.

Tip To prevent blunt shaving, take note of when you start new blades. Depending on the toughness of your beard, replace at regular intervals for a smooth shave.

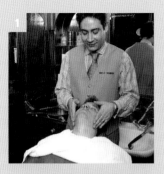
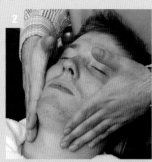
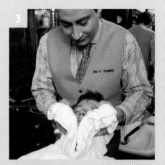
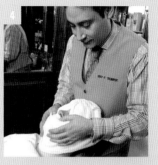
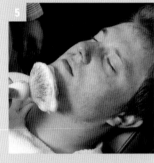
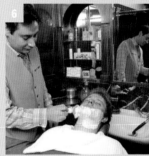
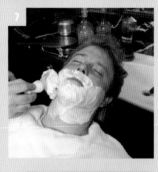
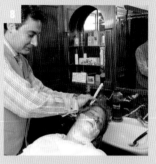
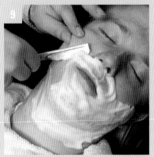
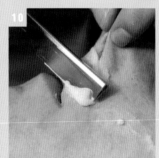
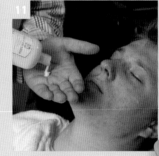
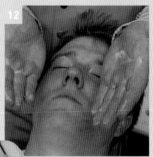

LEARN FROM THE PROFESSIONALS

HOW TO ACHIEVE THE PERFECT SHAVE

(1, 2) Properly prepare the beard area; wet the skin with warm soapy water to start to open the pores and soften the beard. **(3, 4)** Gently dry with a warm towel. **(5, 6, 7)** Using a circular motion, apply shaving gel with your fingers or lather with a brush. Beard hair grows in several directions and by spreading the lather in circles there is less risk of missing an area. In addition, this encourages the beard to spring out from the skin in preparation for the shave. **(8)** Shave in the direction of the hair growth in short easy sweeps, taking your time and feeling the direction of the beard with your fingers. **(9, 10)** Use your fingers to gently pull the skin tighter as you shave across the face, chin, and finally the neck. If need be, re-apply lather and shave again. Check that stray hairs higher up on the cheeks have not been missed and that the sideburns are even, and rinse off any remaining lather with cold water. **(11, 12)** Finally, apply moisturizer to the shaved area.

AFTER SHAVING

After shaving, the pores are open. Cool to ice-cold water splashed over the face will remove the last of the lather, close the pores, and tighten the skin. Since shaving is in effect a daily exfoliation of the surface of the skin, men generally have tougher skin than women, and it needs moisturizing.

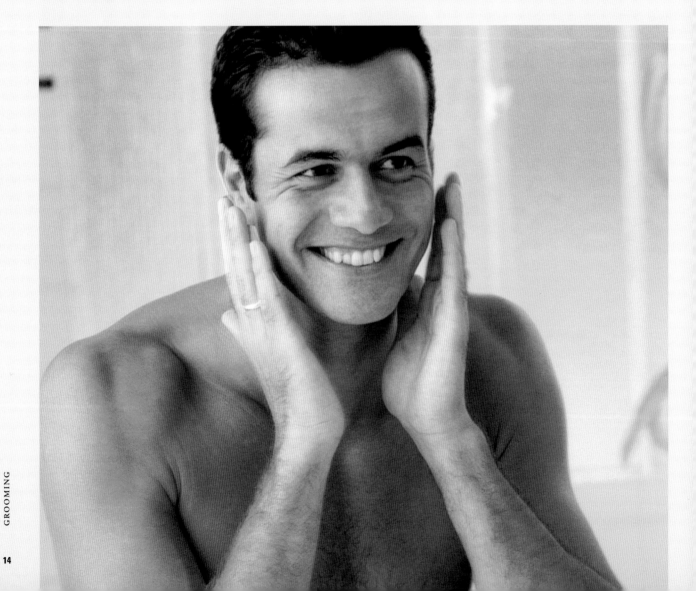

There are many hundreds of skin preparations on the market that are suitable for moisturizing newly shaved skin but there are some easy guidelines to narrow down the options. Your basic skin type is easy to check through simple analysis: dry, oily, combination, or normal. Put simply, does your skin tend to dryness and flaking? Do you have greasy and shiny skin? Are parts of your face dry and others oily, or does your skin seem to function normally with no extreme patches at all?

It is also important to think about the kind of daily routine you keep; whether, for example, you are in air-conditioned and heated environments most of the time, or generally outdoors in all weathers. The combination of your skin type and your lifestyle has an effect on your skin and consequently on the kind of preparation you should be using. Whatever moisturizer you select, it should not sting or smart after shaving but instead provide moisture and protection from the daily onslaught that your skin receives. Your moisturizer should restore moisture to the skin to keep it looking good and retain its elasticity.

Tip *When attending an evening function for which you must leave directly from work, find time to give your face a wash and apply a small drop of moisturizer to freshen up.*

Selecting an after-shave treatment is going to take some time. There are balms, moisturizers, lotions, creams, and liquids to choose from and they vary in price over a wide range. Generally the simple answer is that, whatever the price or brand, the biggest sellers tend to be those that large numbers of men have been satisfied with through a process of trial and error. Many of these products are classics in their field rather than novelties. Trial and error testing in the store, with samples and advice from experts, will carry you through to a successful outcome.

Tip *If your partner already has a trusted skincare consultant, visit with him or her for some advice.*

You may also want to consider other skin products to use after shaving as part of your grooming routine. Eye creams for puffiness or shadows under the eyes, an occasional face mask to cleanse deeper than just soap and water, or even a neck cream for crepey skin. There are, as with moisturizers, literally thousands of specialized preparations available and you should spend time looking and sampling to discover those that suit your needs, lifestyle, and budget.

Left: *Buying treatments from a single company can help avoid skin discomfort and strange scent combinations, which may be caused by mismatched ingredients.*

15

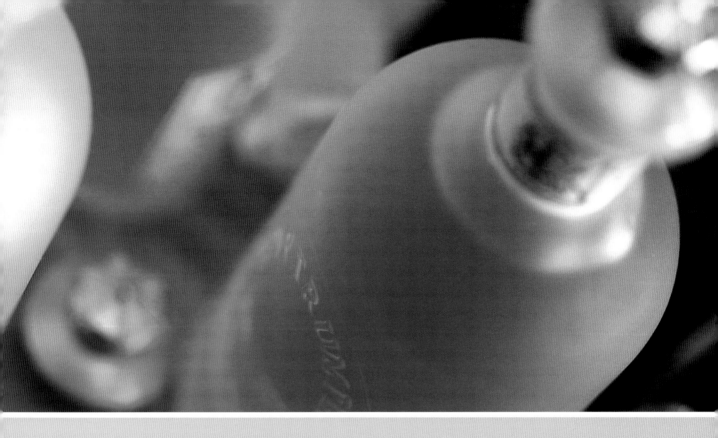

FRAGRANCE

Fragrance for men has a noble history. From ancient Egyptian times it developed into an important part of men's grooming. In eighteenth-century France courtiers at the court of Louis XV were mad about fragrance, while in England in Regency times gentlemen's cologne and toilet water were an accepted part of grooming. Floris in Jermyn Street, London, opened as a barber in 1730 and by 1800 had one hundred specially made fragrances, many of which Beau Brummell must have tried during his frequent visits. The shop is still there, with wonderful mahogany showcases offering some of those same products and displaying the first of many royal warrants granted by George IV when he became King in 1820. Guerlain of Paris, one of the oldest perfume houses in the world, still produces Eau de Cologne Impériale, launched in 1860. The many toilet water and eau de cologne-based men's fragrances available today have a direct lineage from this Guerlain classic.

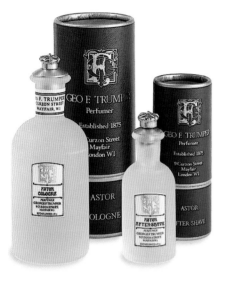

Above: *Classic fragrance from an upscale barber, in apothecary-style bottles, can lift your spirit.*

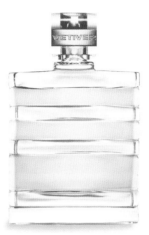

Above: *Guerlain's Vetiver scent in its chunky glass bottle suits a man's bathroom.*

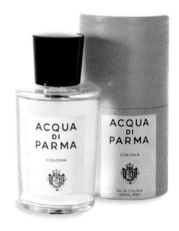

Above: *Old-fashioned scents are the benchmark in men's fragrance and never go out of fashion.*

In the twentieth century, aftershaves and deodorants began to be introduced from the 1950s onward and by the 1970s were an accepted part of a gentleman's life. Many of them are classics which are still available today: Arden for Men (1953, Elizabeth Arden); Pour Monsieur (1955, Chanel); Old Spice (1957, Old Spice); Aramis (1959, Estée Lauder); Vetiver (1959, Guerlain); Eau Sauvage (1964, Christian Dior); Brut (1964, Fabergé); Habit Rouge (1965, Guerlain); Monsieur de Givenchy (1966, Hubert de Givenchy); YSL Pour Homme (1971, Yves Saint Laurent); Gucci Pour Homme (1976, Gucci); Polo for Men (1978, Ralph Lauren).

Tip Test scents on your skin and allow yourself time to discover what suits your skin, what other people respond to, and what lingers at the right level.

Fragrance is like a personal signature, which may change for the occasion and the climate. The cardinal rule for men is: never, ever, be heavily scented. Fragrance may, for example, be sprinkled on a handkerchief, or dabbed and sprayed at pulse points—neck, ears, and wrists. Many fragrances contain oils and coloring, which can leave stains on fabrics, so you should take care with their application. Note also that in a hot climate, a heavy scent will evaporate; it is far better to emulate the Latin male with a series of splashed, eau de toilette, or cologne-style fragrances. These are much more refreshing and may be applied more frequently owing to their lightness.

Tip A man's fragrance, unlike a woman's, should not linger; it is only at close range that the fragrance should become apparent.

If more than one product from a range is used, take care that the accumulated effect is not overwhelming. Another danger area is using a range of toiletries, each of which contains a different fragrance. The combined effect can become eye-watering in its strength.

Consider the appropriate style for the occasion: a sporty splash for weekend use or a sophisticated cologne for a black-tie dinner, for example. Trial and error will lead to some odd discoveries, such as a fragrance that you liked but which fails to stay on your skin for more than a few brief minutes, or certain notes in a fragrance that overwhelm the rest in reaction to your skin.

When you discover the scent that pleases you and those around you, stay with it for a while. Fashion will as always dictate change, but for now you can relax in your choices.

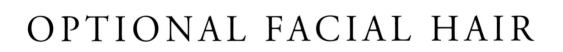

OPTIONAL FACIAL HAIR

When you meet someone for the first time, your face gives them a strong impression of how you present yourself. Nature has given men facial hair that varies with each individual in color, density, and growth; you have to decide how you wish to frame or even decorate your face with facial hair. There are, however, a few rules that should be considered when dealing with this area of grooming.

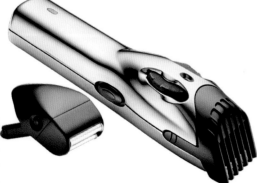

BEARDS, MOUSTACHES, & SIDEBURNS Whatever facial hair you may grow, the golden rule is to keep it groomed. Wild straggly hair, which spells unkempt to the observer, has no place in a gentleman's appearance. A beard may be closely trimmed, Vandyke-style, or a goatee, but it should always be neat and trimmed either by yourself, with the aid of a beard trimmer, or by your barber. The moustache, as one option of facial hair, is very much a victim of the whims of fashion—the pencil-thin moustache of the 1930s or the heavy cowboy-style moustache of the 70s are just two examples of how fashion can affect facial hair. However, the silver

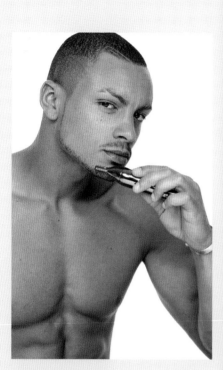

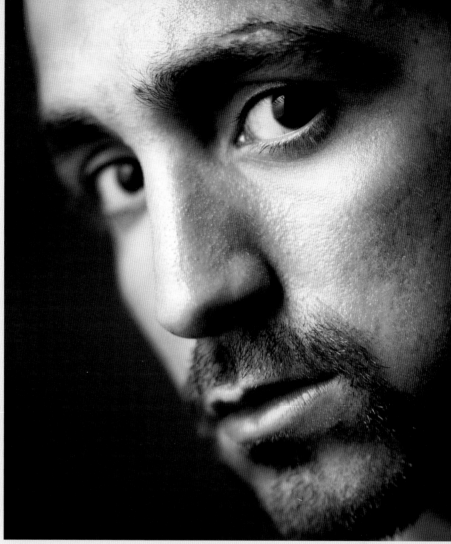

Above and right: *Most men usually require up to six weeks to achieve suitable growth. Whatever your preference—be it a classic goatee or a more flamboyant Vandyke (a pointed trimmed beard with a shaped moustache)—the cardinal rule for a gentleman is to keep facial hair neatly trimmed and spotlessly clean.*

screen style is certainly a classic and vintage option. Since this immaculately groomed variation of facial hair references the past, it is timeless and less likely to be the victim of a sudden change in current style. Other moustache shapes from Hollywood include waxed and curled moustaches either alone—in the manner of Agatha Christie's detective Hercule Poirot—or with a goatee beard in the style of Cardinal Richelieu. The point to be made clear here is that a gentleman adopting any of these variations is making a strong style statement, but one rooted firmly in the past. This does

not prevent this genre of moustache being dashing, imposing, or romantic, it is an option entirely open to a gentleman, should he so choose. This fashion statement also applies to sideburns.

Tip *Stubble is not always rough and sexy; it can also be aging and rather grubby looking. Check which effect your stubble produces before venturing out.*

Keep all facial hair spotlessly clean and, as with all hair, free from dryness and flaking. Specialized preparations are available to treat these conditions, but regular washing and moisturizing should generally be all that is required. Since all facial hair makes a personal statement, make certain that your facial hair is saying the correct thing about you and your style.

Tip *Hair color on the head and face may vary in tone, or sometimes shade; make certain that any facial hair is flattering and not scruffy or aging.*

FACIAL HAIR

Stray hair growth can be unflattering, either by creating unsightly outlines on the face or adversely affecting the impression one makes on others. Sideburns that are uneven or exaggerated in shape, over-luxuriant eyebrows, and fur-covered ears will do nothing to improve your features. Consider the close scrutiny of your facial hair as part of your grooming ritual and you will be surprised at the confidence which this extra attention to detail will bring to your overall day-to-day life. A gentleman should be secure in the knowledge that, even in close contact with others, he is well groomed—and this includes hair in the ears, nose, and eyebrows. Time spent on detail, rather than getting used to a rushed and cursory facial routine, can only be beneficial—do not think that people will not notice.

Right: Be very careful when trimming or plucking facial hair: do not remove too much. If you do nothing else, trim or pluck the hair from between the brows to avoid looking like a Neanderthal. If you would like a cleaner look, you can also trim any straggling hairs above the brow line, but do not touch the brow's arch.

EYEBROWS In recent years, people have come to realize that a man's eyebrows may not naturally grow in a neat and tidy manner. There are many methods for controlling the line and shape, thus preventing the untidy and menacing monobrow or diabolical tufts shooting across your forehead. The only advice to be remembered is that a man's eyebrows are thicker by nature and less defined than a woman's. Too perfect, too arched, or too waxed are both unattractive and unmanly.

Tip It is essential when working on facial hair to have excellent light and, ideally, a magnifying mirror.

EARS AND NOSE As men grow older, body hair often increases, although some men are generally more hairy than others. Hairy ears should be plucked, waxed, or treated. Nose hairs should be neatly trimmed with nail scissors to prevent any unsightly fringe effect. It is very important to remember that nasal hairs are there for a purpose and to remove them too heavily, thus exposing the nasal cavity, is both uncomfortable and unhealthy.

Tip Keep all tweezers and trimmers spotlessly clean and always replace them at regular intervals.

Right: *Remember that, whatever hair-removal regimen you choose to follow, it fits with your lifestyle. Do not choose a high-maintenance look if your morning schedule does not allow it. This will result in an unattended and scruffy look, and is entirely avoidable.*

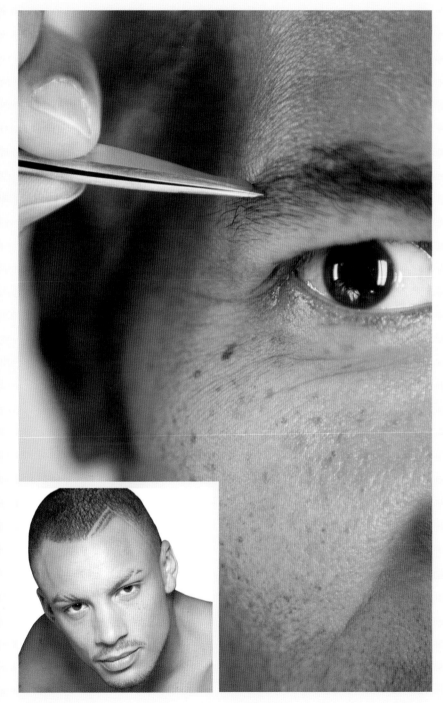

YOU & YOUR BARBER

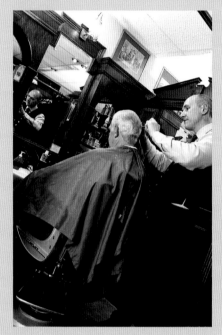

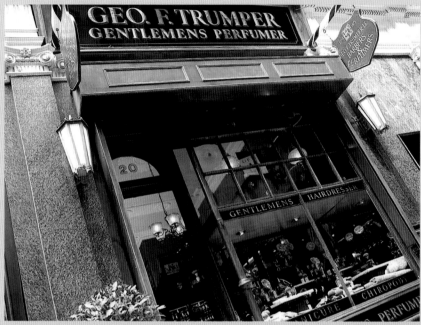

There is a hairstyle to suit everyone. Hair may be floppy and straight, springy and curly, or thinning; you may have a double crown, or salt and pepper hair that requires discreet coloring—any kind of hair will benefit from a good cut and professional advice.

Your barber or hairdresser should advise and support you in the same way as your dentist or optician. Since your hair frames your face, a bad or incorrect haircut can fatten, elongate, or broaden your features. It may also date you with an old-fashioned cut or simply fail to match your lifestyle. You may know what you like or want from a haircut, but your hairdresser or barber must also give an opinion, and should never let you leave looking less than your best.

Tip *Bear in mind that the most fashionable hairstyle of the moment will, like the layered and permed styles of the 80s, eventually go out of style and, if retained, will date you.*

There is also the important matter of the health of your hair: dandruff, split ends, and dryness must be dealt with effectively. Nothing creates a worse impression than a sprinkling of scalp flakes across the shoulders of a dark suit. The role of the hair salon within your life is an important one.

Skincare at barber shops and salons has expanded in recent years, but traditional hot towel treatments and the trimming of ear hair have always been acceptable for even the least vain man. If your salon offers spa treatments, pedicures as well as manicures, or any other body maintenance, consider availing yourself of the facilities.

HAIRSTYLES

HOW TO WEAR YOUR HAIR

CLASSIC/SCHOOLBOY/SHORT BACK AND SIDES This is the haircut that is tapered from the crown to the ears and nape with a side parting and a fringe. It is never out of fashion, but is not a statement hairstyle; however, for many men in business this style works well because the fringe may be gelled back for work and left floppy for weekends, thus proving its surprising versatility, hence its longevity.

SPIKED Originally called "Hoxton Fin" after the area of London where it was first most fashionable, this style has developed into a mainstream obsession in recent years. Requiring a layered cut and a great deal of product to achieve a lasting series of spikes or peaks, this style is best left to those with a luxuriant head of hair and a great deal of patience. It is nowhere near as easy to achieve as its disheveled appearance would lead you to believe.

SHAVED For many men, once hair loss has been accepted, or in the case of wild unmanageable hair, shaving is a great option. This may be done at home, but there are also many men who from time to time want a hairdresser to treat the scalp or give a massage to make certain they are as well-groomed as their hirsute companions.

CROPPED OR CREW CUT The crop is defined by the blades used for the cut, with number 1 being the shortest. The crop may use two or three numbers for less severity, but it is neat, easy, masculine, and ideal for thinning hair. The style is also excellent if you lead a busy life with many different roles, including sports activities. It can be washed in the shower and requires minimal maintenance between cuts.

LONG HAIR The first major factor in deciding to have long hair is having quality hair. Then you must be prepared to maintain your hair in peak condition. Long hair may be jaw-length, shoulder-length, or even longer, but it must always be well cut and trimmed, spotlessly clean, and, in many business environments, tied back neatly. Above all, hair should never be long if it is thinning, wildly unmanageable, or fine and straggly.

BALDNESS Although we all hope that it will not happen to us, for many the day dawns when you can no longer ignore the thinning signs across the forehead or on the crown of your head. This is the time to decide how you are going to cope with the situation. Shaved, number-1 crop, a neat short back and sides, or even a slight touch of Caesar with the hair short but brushed and gelled forward: all of these styles are acceptable; what is not acceptable is a comb-over, a bad toupée, or any other sign of non-acceptance of the situation.

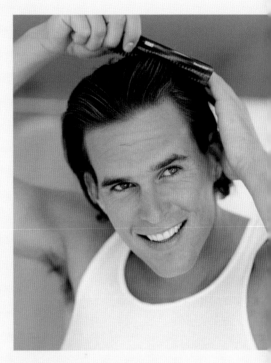

Above: Whether worn long, short, or very closely cropped, hair must be kept neat and tidy. Regular visits to the barber should be part of a gentleman's routine.

HAIR PRODUCTS

Most hairdressers are affiliated with certain products and promote them to their customers. These products will generally be made by the major players within the industry and as such will be reliable; in addition, salon staff will be informed of the latest developments and trends.

Hair mousse, hair gel, hair wax, and so on, have all been developed in response to the ever-changing needs of style. The traditional haircut has long been superseded by wash, color, cut, and blow dry; hair straighteners may now be added to this list. At home you will have a range of products in addition to a hairdryer, brushes, and combs to reproduce the effects on a day-to-day basis.

Right and below: *Whatever hair product you select, ensure it is suitable for your hair type and style. If you choose not to use product on your hair, be sure to tell your barber or hairdresser, and choose a cut that will work without product, but don't be quick to go without. Pomade, for example, is a great all-rounder if you have thick and curly hair that tends to be frizzy.*

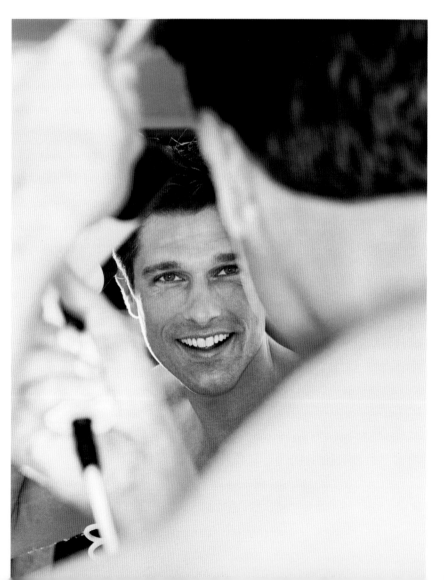

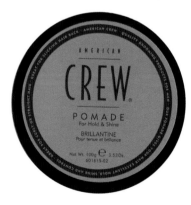

SHAMPOO & CONDITIONER

There are hundreds of shampoos and conditioners available for the cleanliness and care of the hair. Aside from those recommended and used by your barber or hairdresser, you may have specific brands whose other products you already use, gifts from partners and friends, or new products you are thinking of trying. The basic formulas may vary and there is always the risk that a particular product will not suit your hair type, skin, or scalp. If a shampoo or conditioner disagrees with you, throw it out, wait for the condition it has caused to die down, and then try a new shampoo. Baby shampoos are often effective in combating the after-effects of an abrasive shampoo or conditioner.

Tip It is not advisable to buy conditioner and shampoo in one; they are doing separate jobs and should come in separate containers.

Hair products such as wax or gel may cause an allergic reaction or excessive drying of the hair, as may overuse of the hairdryer. These reactions may not always be immediate; they often result from long-term use and can usually be avoided by switching products from time to time.

Tip When choosing a hairdresser, it is of great importance to seek out someone who understands your personality and lifestyle as well as your personal idiosyncrasies.

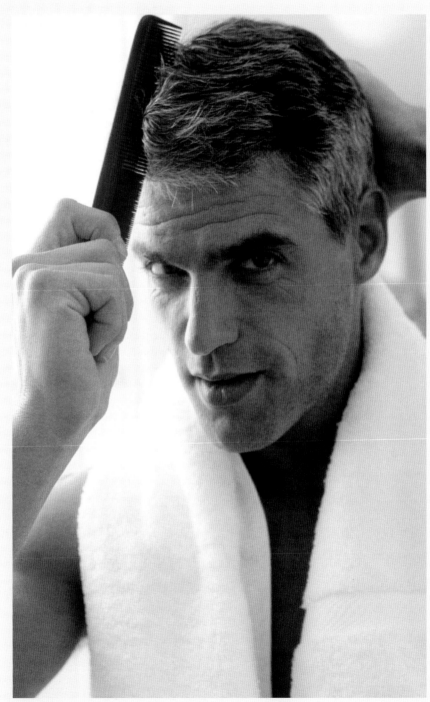

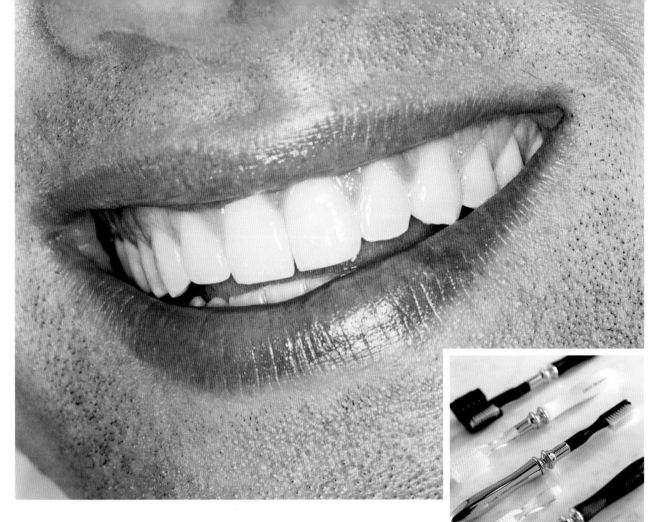

TEETH & BREATH

Your dentist is a vital member of your grooming team and, as such, should be chosen for his professional know-how, ease of access (there is no point in having a dentist several miles away), and reliability. There are, in today's world, staggering arrays of cosmetic treatments available within dentistry. Many of these are well worth the investment to provide you with healthy, well-shaped teeth, and a confident smile. Since many procedures are constantly being updated or introduced, it is important to question your dentist about these innovations, and their possible application to you. The shape, evenness, and color of your teeth should be considered part of your overall grooming program.

Regular visits to your dentist are the simple answer to dental care. If teeth are cared for and maintained throughout your life, there should be little cause for concern or the development of unexpected trouble.

CLEANING Always make time to clean your teeth, thus giving them the maximum help in being healthy and lasting. Carrying toothbrush and toothpaste whenever possible means you can give your teeth a clean when the opportunity or the need arises, whatever form your regular cleaning procedure takes.

SHAPE There are now many variations of cosmetic dentistry to correct uneven teeth and create a more harmonious shape. Procedures have been developed which, although expensive, will, in the long term, give you greater confidence. The key role of all dental work is to enable you to feel that, while communicating with those around you, there is nothing to for you to be concerned about.

COLOR Although there are many tooth-whitening toothpastes and solutions, there is no substitute for professional expertise. The whiteness of teeth has become a major concern to most men in recent years. Dental work to create the correct form of natural-appearing whiteness and evenness is a job for an expert—and can go badly wrong if done at home.

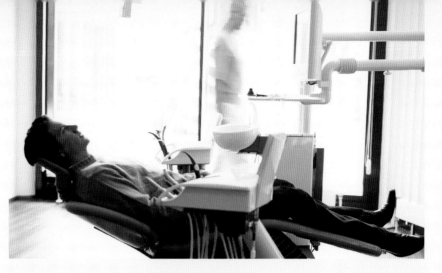

Above: Dental care at home is no substitute for visiting the dentist. And be wary of bleaching your teeth: bright, optical white teeth can make you look like a game-show host.

BREATH Bad breath may be traced either to teeth or to diet and stomach problems. In either case, it must be dealt with through the appropriate treatment. Regular use of mouthwash is vital, and mouth fresheners are now available in handy formats from sprays to individual leaves. Keep a toothbrush and toothpaste at work for after lunch, pre-meeting, or post-work freshness.

Tip Take care that peppermint-flavored breath is not overwhelming for your colleagues. Wait 20 minutes before a meeting after you've used strong mints.

LIPS Chapped, dry, cracked, or sore lips can be the result of many things, from nerves to exposure to harsh elements through sports. In any event, they are both uncomfortable and unattractive. Lip balms and salves come in a wide range: slim tubes, sticks, and small tins. They take up no room in either a pocket or case ready for application at any time they are needed. The one thing to remember is that the intention is to keep the lips moist and clean, not to provide a shine.

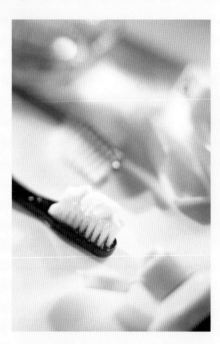

Note on equipment Electric toothbrushes, dental floss, tooth powders, and so on, should all be discussed with the expert who tends to your teeth. You may damage as much as cleanse with the incorrect equipment.

Tip Always read articles on new dental procedures, treatments, and products to decide if you wish to inquire further.

HANDS

First impressions count
and your hands can say a
tremendous amount about you.
Caring for your hands is not a question
of vanity or fussiness, it is common sense.
Boardroom or factory, dinner table or diner,
your hands are much in evidence at work or at
leisure and are able to communicate a great deal
about your approach to life. Above all, they are
vital tools in your day-to-day existence for every
business and leisure activity.

SKINCARE Sitting all day at a desk may seem far less harmful to your hands than straightforward manual work, but at all times and in all situations your hands are exposed to dryness, minor cuts and bruises, pollution, and many other influences. Washing your hands regularly is good, but restoring some moisture is also essential. Hand cream comes in a wide range of formulas and containers; choose one that suits your lifestyle and use it regularly to both nourish and protect your hands.

Tip *When you wash your hands, the cuticles are softened, so push them gently back with the towel as you dry your hands.*

NAILS Use nail clippers or scissors for cutting the nail and an emery board to smooth the top edge. A soft cuticle stick can be used to gently push the cuticle back; under no circumstances should you ever cut the cuticle, which is a natural buffer against infection under the nail bed. For a man, the nail should be trimmed short, curved to reflect the shape of the top of the finger, with the cuticles well pushed back and the surface clean and buffed. An over-manicured hand, with overly polished or shined nails or nails that are too long, simply implies that here is a man who is vain, lazy, and afraid of getting his hands dirty in work or leisure.

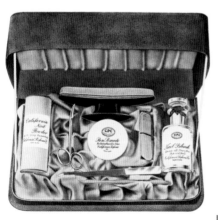

Above: *A grooming kit for hands and nails is a sound investment, but simply keeping your cuticles moisturized and nails clipped will make a dramatic difference.*

NAIL HEALTH The health of a man can often be diagnosed by the health of his nails, which may be attributed to diet or to a medical condition. If you have splitting nails, heavily ridged nails, or some other problem with your nails, it is important not to ignore it but to deal with the problem immediately—consult your physician.

Tip Money invested in appropriate gloves is money well spent, since gloves protect your hands in bad weather conditions as well as during some sports.

MANICURES A manicure has long been an accepted part of a man's grooming ritual. Many barbers or hairdressers provide a manicurist though not all are equally good, and it is better to go elsewhere if you regularly need a good manicure. Women have many salons that offer nail treatments, but not all are equally expert at men's manicures, so make sure they have a regular clientele of satisfied male customers before you put your hands in theirs.

EXERCISE Stretching and flexing your hand and fingers, especially after a long bout of repetitive work, is a good idea. Sitting at a computer for several hours, or any activity at which the same movements are performed over again and again means that the hands will likely feel tired. Putting your hands high in the air and then flexing your fingers stimulates the circulation and the muscles.

HAND CARE
SIMPLE STEPS FOR WELL-GROOMED HANDS

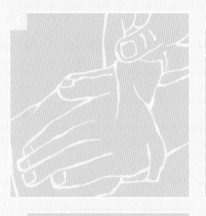

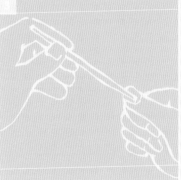

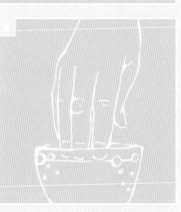

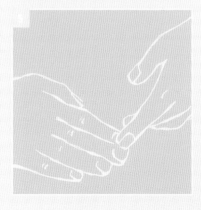

(1) Wear latex gloves for manual jobs to protect your skin and nails from dirt and chemicals. Use an emery board to keep nail ends smooth and less likely to split. **(2)** Lightly buff the nail to reduce ridges. **(3)** Only use a soft implement to push back the cuticles and never cut them. **(4)** Soften your nails in warm water before trimming them with scissors or clippers. **(5)** Finally, moisturize your nails as well as your skin. Cuticle cream will prevent your cuticles from becoming rough and cracking.

FEET

Your feet bear the full weight of your body as well as providing you with motion. Problems with your feet will make life extremely difficult for you, so it is therefore a sound investment to spend time and trouble on them to avoid such an eventuality. Before you even put shoes on, or contemplate a chiropodist for a pedicure and foot treatment, you should be doing your best to look after your feet yourself.

SKIN Your feet are possibly the hardest-working part of your body, in every sense, and therefore they develop rough and hard skin very easily. This must be treated regularly and not be allowed to build up. Softening and soaking the feet will help, as will using a file or pumice stone on extra-tough skin, but professional help is often the best solution, along with good maintenance between visits. All areas of the foot are vulnerable to athlete's foot, from beneath the toes to the heels, but regular washing followed by some type of moisturizer will help to keep this condition at bay. Always dry carefully between the toes and keep feet dry since dampness leads to problem conditions. Bunions, corns, and other problem conditions must be dealt with by a professional as soon as they appear.

NAILS Toenails should be regularly trimmed and kept very short; this is easy to do with the correct clippers. Pedicures will supplement the day-to-day care of your toenails and will also indicate if there are any areas that need treatment for ingrowing, splitting, or other toenail problems.

EXERCISE Exercise for the feet is vital since, like all working parts, they need to be flexed or they will develop problems. This is especially true when traveling or working in a sedentary job.

HOLIDAY FEET Vacation is the time your feet are most open to scrutiny, but this is also the time they will, hopefully, be at their healthiest. Walking barefoot on sand gently erodes dry skin while the toes and instep are being flexed and exercised; even beach sandals and flip-flops make the feet work harder. Lightly tanned feet are attractive, but take the same precautions with sunscreen on your feet as on any other part of the body. Sunburned feet are agony!

SPORTS FEET For all forms of sport and exercise it is of prime importance to wear the correct shoes to support and protect the feet. The stress placed on your feet by many sports and activities means that they are especially vulnerable to problems. It therefore makes sense to treat your feet well during and after all sporting activities.

Tip If your feet have a tendency to sweat, wear lightweight socks and change them frequently.

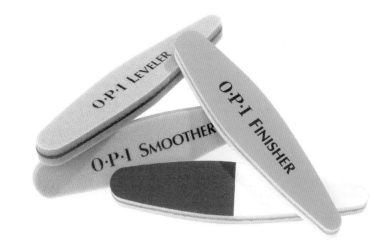

LIFESTYLE Vary your footwear according to the situation; if you wear a solid business shoe all day, change into a slipper or lightweight shoe at home. It is good for your feet to have a range of shoe types; changing shoes more frequently prolongs the life of the shoe and also demonstrates your understanding of the appropriate footwear for different occasions.

Tip After an exhausting day or a long journey, lie flat on your back with your legs and feet up in the air (against a wall is easiest) to ease swollen ankles or insteps.

Note If you have major foot odor problems, seek professional advice.

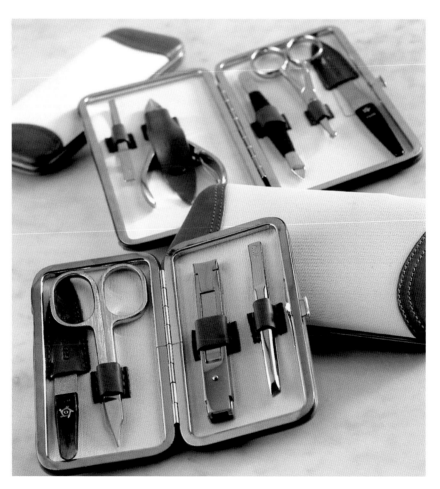

Right: Feet are vital to health, fitness, and comfort in daily life and should never be neglected. A man's pedicure kit will keep your feet looking their best.

BODY (1)

The body is often described as a machine and, like any good machine, to function best it needs constant maintenance. You must consider the needs of the inside and the outside of your body in order to benefit from all that life offers you. After all, a tired and stressed body with many small imperfections will not sustain a happy, active, and motivated life.

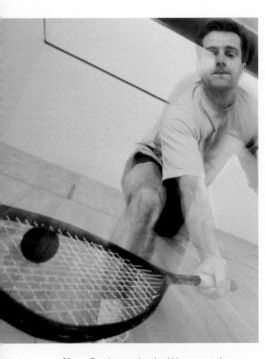

Above: *Regular exercise should become routine— three times a week is recommended—rather than in intense but sporadic outbursts, which are so often subsequently dropped.*

EXERCISE There are several options for exercising, each of which suits a different lifestyle and personality. Membership at a local gym with instructors and flexible hours is one method. Home gyms are a great idea if you have the space, but you must have the motivation to regularly use the facilities to their full benefit. Another home option is a personal trainer who will advise you on what equipment to invest in for the correct results. There are many other activities for keeping fit, such as running, and team sports. With all these variations there are two overriding factors to take into account. The first is to stick to whatever form of exercise you select—taking out annual membership at a gym in January and then never using it after March is a big waste of time and money. Second, get help and support in the form of instructors and someone to train and exercise with. Unless you are very committed it is a great help to have competition and someone to push you when you are slacking.

DIET What you put into your body certainly has an effect on the way your body responds and behaves. Diet is reflected in your weight, energy, and every part of your body from your hair down to your toenails. Doctors and dieticians can support and correct your diet where there are specific problems and allergies, but you must start by having respect for your body in what you choose to put into it. Common sense and some thought can often help you analyze why you are either lethargic or putting on weight, and a bit of adjustment to your day-to-day diet can often result in some surprisingly effective outcomes. Crash diets are a waste of time since it is only through consistency and maintenance that the body will respond and stay healthy.

Tip A fad or fashionable diet is exactly that: a fad or a fashion. There is no substitute for sensible, healthy eating.

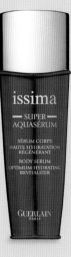

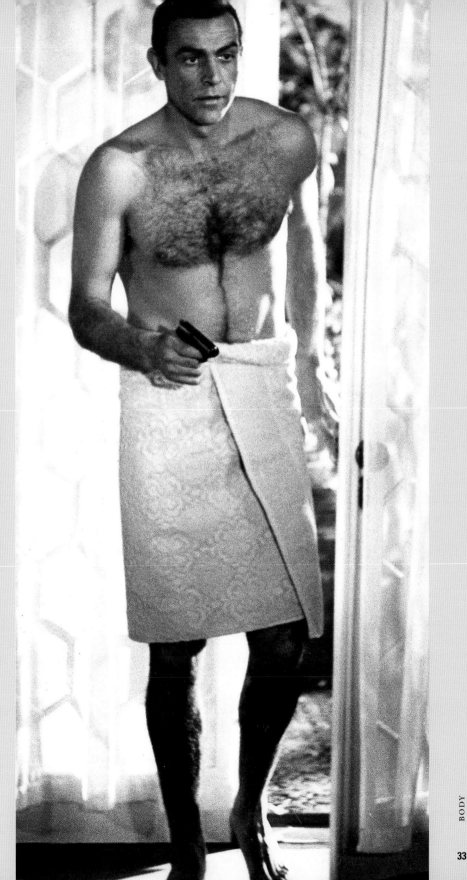

Right: *Sean Connery, here playing James Bond, demonstrates that a man's body hair is a sign of virility at any age.* **Left:** *A body moisturizer will soothe the skin and help prevent signs of premature aging.*

SKIN The largest organ of the body is your skin, so it surely makes sense to look after it. If you are healthy and fit, your skin should reflect this, but the skin also requires maintenance just as the body of a car does. Check over your body at regular intervals to note any skin discolorations, bruising, or other changes which might need checking out by a physician or dermatologist. The skin on your body may have areas of dryness and areas that receive harder work than others—for example, elbows—tend to get dry and need extra moisture. Cleansers like soap and shower gel, deodorants, and bath and shower preparations all support the presentation of your skin. Using an all-over body moisturizer after you get out of the shower will help seal in the moisture.

Tip Change deodorants occasionally since from time to time the body either becomes used to them or perhaps reacts against them.

BODY (2)

The care of your body will encompass both nature and art. Nature generally gives men body hair, which must be considered as part of your grooming program; and you may employ artistry in the matter of body decoration, from a temporary tattoo through body piercing. It is for each individual to make his own decisions.

BODY HAIR Stray hairs should be neatly plucked out with tweezers, and any major hair removal should be done by a professional using waxing or another appropriate method, such as electrolysis. Untidy or overabundant body hair may also be neatened with electric clippers. However, body hair is very much a personal matter, to be considered along with the feelings of your partner. Waxing a variety of parts of the body from the chest downward has become fashionable for men in recent years; again, the choice is personal.

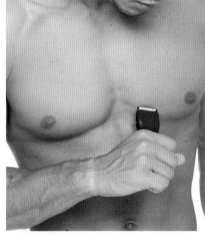

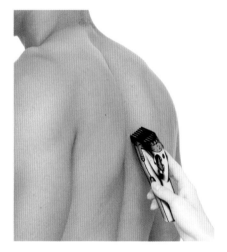

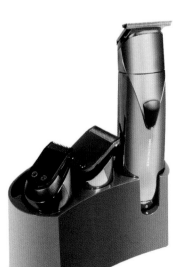

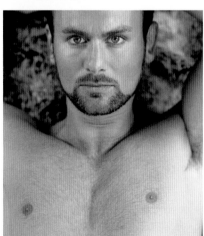

Above and left: Once confined to competitive athletes such as body builders and swimmers, male body hair removal has become more popular in the past few years. Neat body hair or totally shaved is a personal and partner choice. If you do choose to remove body hair, note that waxing will last longer than shaving, but can be quite painful. If you choose to shave, you will have to do it more frequently, and stubble can be uncomfortable. Vigilant use of an exfoliating scrub will help prevent ingrowing hairs and razor bumps, and a thick moisturizer will help ease skin, which may dry out after shaving.

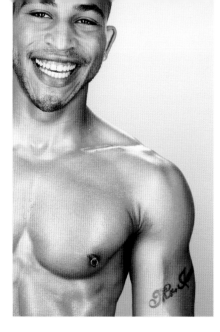

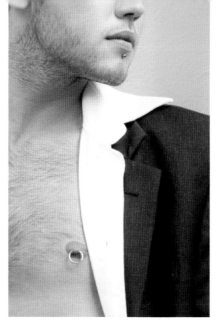

Left: Tattoos and/or piercings are intimate expressions of style and, for most lifestyles, are best kept discreet.

TATTOOS Sadly, tattoos are as subject to fashion as any other style element. The best advice regarding tattoos is to make certain that they can be covered up part of the time. Biceps tattoos that may be hidden by T-shirt sleeves, and discreet motifs on the back, thighs, and chest work well since they need not be visible in an inappropriate situation. Remember, as you age and your skin loses its firmness, the tattoo will lose its impact. In addition, the ink will gently fade with time, so the tattoo will not remain as it is but will age with you. It is important to have a tattoo done only at a hygienic and recommended tattoo parlor.

Tip *Have a full-length mirror in your bathroom and, if possible, another one positioned to enable you to view yourself from all angles.*

PIERCING Eyebrows, lips, and tongue are all highly visible places for piercing, and thus signal how you define your image. There are many professionals in which this is not a problem, but before having a visible piercing, make absolutely sure it will not impair your career progress. Once again, fashion has a surprisingly strong influence on piercing. Where once many men viewed a pierced ear as the height of

unconventionality, we now see this as a little unstylish and outdated. Any piercing should be kept scrupulously clean at all times. If you decide to undergo any type of piercing, make certain the person doing it has a good reputation. Be sure to ask about the possibility of temporary piercing. Consider the consequences of removal and scarring or healing if you later decide to permanently remove the piercing.

MOLES If you have moles anywhere on your body, make sure they are checked out by a dermatologist or doctor at regular intervals. Also monitor them yourself and watch for any changes in color, shape, or size. Sunbathing and exposure may especially affect moles on the body.

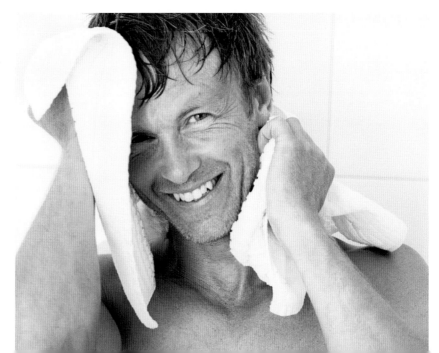

Right: Make sure you dry yourself completely after a shower or bath. Damp skin can cause irritation, especially between the toes or under the arms.

BODY (3)

The body, once in good physical condition, may be pampered; this is not entirely for sybaritic reasons, but also for the general health and well-being of its owner. Relaxation through body maintenance and the general care of the skin is the perfect antidote to the cares and stresses of everyday life, both professional and domestic. The results of looking after your body include enhancement of leisure time, better sleep, and renewed energy.

SHOWERS Showers are a part of the day-to-day life of millions of people on this planet. Especially in preparation for the daily routine, and that includes work, the speed with which you may take a shower is a great asset. Your shower should be well-stocked with everything you need. There is nothing less conducive to a gentleman's good temper than a shower that needs turning as though one were cracking a safe, towels out of reach, and cheap containers of generic shampoo and liquid soap.

Get your shower fixed so there is a decent flow of water at the correct temperature, buy new towels to hang within easy reach of the shower, and finally invest in some decent products to be placed in a convenient shower rack that hangs in the shower stall itself. Make sure that after shampooing and soaping you remove all foam and suds before stepping out of the shower, since the residue will do nothing for the health of your skin.

Tip If speed is of the essence when showering before going out in the evening, keep the water cool to cold for maximum effect.

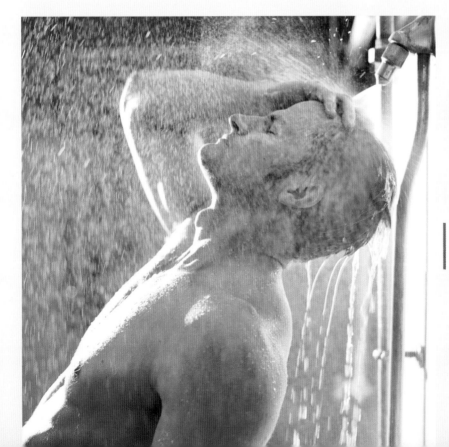

Left: *Consider installing a shower filter if your water is highly chlorinated. Chlorinated water can dry out your skin and decrease the air quality in your home.*

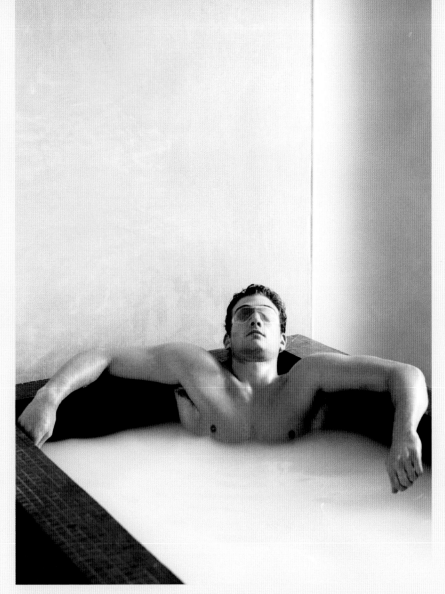

SPA If your shower and bath at home are not enough, there are now more and more spa centers to choose from that help to pamper, restore, or invigorate the body. It is important to decide what you are looking for and what is going to benefit your body. Health farms and spas often overlap in their offerings of diet, treatments, and exercise. Specialized treatments are also available, depending in many cases on what products are preferred by the spa and also on what part of the world they are in, relative to natural resources such as mud baths, hot springs, and other locally available body treatments. Your visit can vary from one day to a week; there are even some spa concepts that allow a short visit for scalp massage and skin treatment. The developments in this area of grooming are ever-growing and it is important to balance personal preferences with the newly fashionable, since not all treatments are effective for men.

THE BATH If you do not have a bathtub at home, it is important to take advantage when you do have access to one, perhaps at a hotel. After work, before bed, when stressed, or simply as a pick-me-up before a party, the slow pampering of a bath is special. Scented and moisturizing potions may be added to the water, and special soaps mean that each area of the body may be massaged and treated as you work your way lathering from neck to toes. At night relaxing oil or salts added to the bathwater will ease muscles and induce sleep; candlelit bathrooms create a soporific atmosphere to add to the effect.

Tip *Try to find out what type of mineral content is in the water in the area in which you live so that, if necessary, you can balance it with the products you buy.*

Right: Hot stone therapy encourages relaxation.

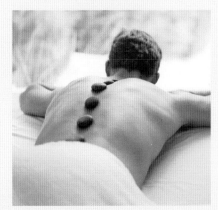

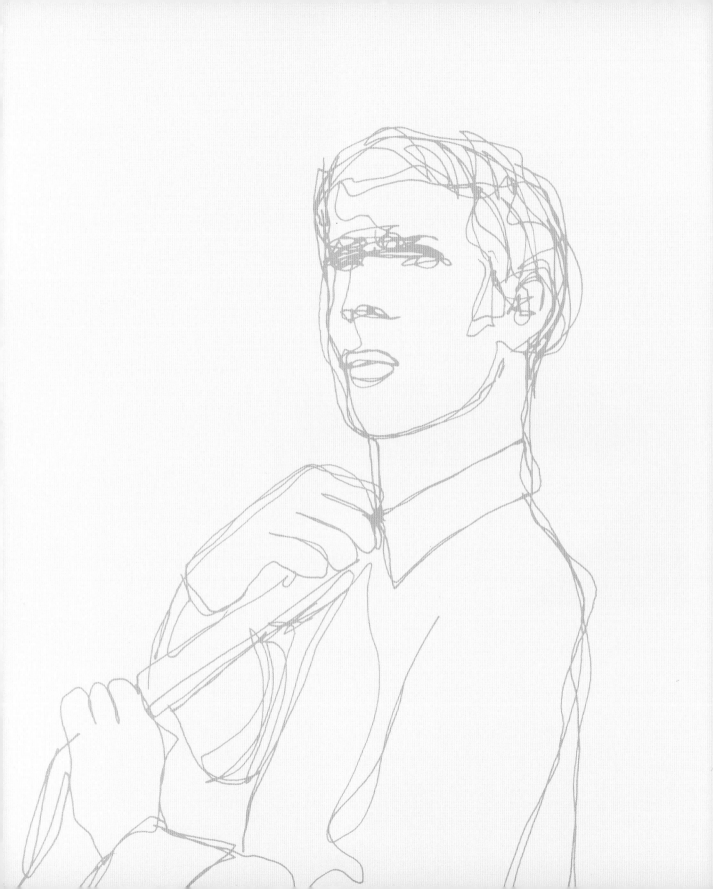

"I realized that I would like to design my own fashion when I saw for myself what the market had to offer—rigid and uncomfortable men's suits, without any research in the fabrics, full of conformism and lacking any personal style."

GIORGIO ARMANI, ITALIAN MENSWEAR DESIGNER

ANATOMY OF A SUIT

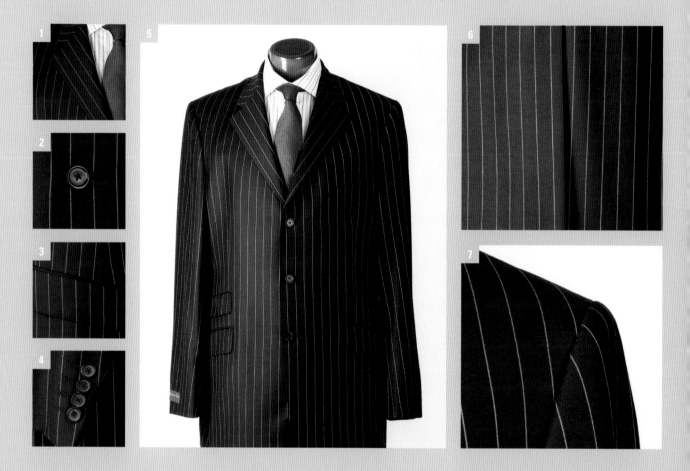

NAMING THE PARTS

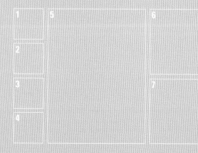

1 The lapel or revers is the fold-back of the lower collar. The size and shape of this design element in a suit plays a key role in the overall effect of style and proportion. (See also fig 7)

2 Buttons should always be in harmony with the fabric and style of the suit.

3 Pockets, whatever the style, should lie flat and flush with the body of the jacket to keep a clean line.

4 Cuff buttons may vary in number but for top quality should actually fasten.

5 The lines and shape of a jacket should be clean and strong, creating an overall impression of masculinity, strength, and perfect grooming.

6 Vents or pleats at the back of a jacket must hang flat and closed, never open or swinging out at an angle.

7 The shoulder line and set of the sleeve should be clean and strong, but never exaggerated.

The purchase of a suit or formal jacket can be time consuming, but when you prepare for the day or occasion and your reflection shows that your style and grooming are successful, it will have been time well spent. All the components of the suit must be considered to achieve this success.

COLLAR The lapel of a jacket may change over several seasons according to fashion. The sharpness, proportion, and angle of the collar are in proportion to the shoulder width and the number of buttons. The length of the jacket also plays a part in the overall balance. When you try on a jacket, check how the collar lies—it should be flat and sharp at the front, curving round to the back of the neck in a neat arc. If it isn't, the collar is incorrectly cut and made, or the fit at the neck is wrong.

SLEEVES The sleeves of a well-cut jacket should never be out of proportion to the shoulder and lapel. Thus, if the shoulder is narrow, it should be accompanied by a slim sleeve; if the fit is easy, a softly cut sleeve is appropriate. Look sideways into the mirror when trying a jacket—the sleeve should fall in a neat gentle curve from the shoulder. Wrinkles or pulling mean the fit is incorrect.

CUFFS On a well-made jacket, the cuffs will have functional buttons so that the cuffs can be folded back for work if required. There will be one, two, three, or four buttons at the cuff; they may vary with one larger and two or three smaller buttons. A cutting-edge jacket may have

more, perhaps as many as six. The cuff of a tailored jacket will flare slightly to accommodate the French cuff of a shirt.

BUTTONS Plain buttons, in matching or tonal colors with a ridge or band around the edge, are timeless. Designer buttons with initials or logos should be discreet and only evident up close. A buttonhole on the lapel is optional, allowing for a boutonnière and, in some cases, a corresponding button on the back of the opposite lapel, so that the wearer may fold the lapels across.

VENTS Vents are the openings at the back of a jacket. There may be a single center vent or a pair either side. Vents should always remain flat and closed when the jacket is buttoned. Their length will vary in relation to the length of the jacket, but should stop at the waist or slightly below.

POCKETS Jacket pockets are not truly designed for fully practical use since the line and fit of a well-cut jacket is distorted by bulging pockets. Furthermore, repeated use stretches the suit fabric. Pockets may be patch (sewn onto the jacket) for a casual look or jetted (inserted into the body of the jacket with a separate flap over the opening)

for formal and business wear. A breast pocket will generally be a patch pocket.

TROUSERS Since trousers suffer more wear and tear than the jacket of a suit, a second pair of trousers may be purchased or ordered. In style, trousers should be in harmony with the jacket, following the silhouette: with a narrow, fitted jacket a slim trouser is appropriate; with an easier fit, choose a straight-legged trouser. Fashion influences trouser details, such as cuffed hems, pleat front styles, or statement shapes such as boot cut or flared. If you are buying a quality suit for long-term use, keep an eye on trendsetting dressers, men's style publications, and Internet fashion news to incorporate only the classic elements that will remain versatile in the long term.

JACKET LENGTHS A simple rule is that a long jacket foreshortens the silhouette by showing less of the trouser. This, in theory, means a tall man is able to wear a longer jacket. However, this does not take into account individual proportions and you may in fact have a long upper body with short legs. Try on several lengths of jacket and study them in the mirror to ascertain the correct length for your body shape.

THE BASICS OF FITTING A SUIT

Purchasing a suit requires time and planning. Check your wardrobe to see what has to be replaced, or what you actually need, and be prepared to try different styles, colors, and fabrics before making your selection.

JACKET

SILHOUETTE The silhouette of a suit starts with the fit and shape. Classic suits are cut fairly lean—a slim body shape, neatly cut armhole and sleeve, is the most flattering. A jacket should fit the body with no distortion or pulling of the fabric when buttoned. Check the fit across the back for wrinkling or excess fabric, and make sure the top of the sleeve and the top of your shoulder are in line. A suit is constructed from the shoulder, collar, and sleeves to give the shape, hang, and fit of the jacket, which then influence the style of trousers.

SHOULDER WIDTH A well-tailored suit should fit across your shoulders, even if the fashion is for an extra narrow fit or a broad padded shoulder.

SINGLE-BREASTED This is the basis of all style variations for the classic suit with buttoning down the center of the jacket.

Options start with a single button at the waist. The two-button style has one at the waist, the second lower down, generally unfastened. Next is three buttons: a waist button and one either side. Four buttons has two above the waist button and one below. The length also influences buttoning, lapel size, and shape. A jacket is all about harmony of proportions and, while a designer jacket may seem to break the rules, if the proportions are pleasing the style will succeed. If the buttoning is wrong, the jacket will neither fit nor hang correctly.

DOUBLE-BREASTED Button two and show four or button four and show six are the usual rules and the buttons are traditionally arranged with wider spacing for the unfastened buttons. Military-style jackets may have several more buttons in straight pairs, all of which fasten.

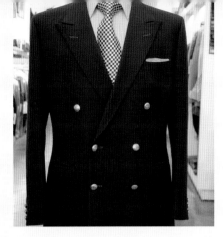

Above: Contrast buttons define this double-breasted jacket as a sporty blazer.
Left: You can't go wrong in business in a single-breasted classic suit.

Tip Double-breasted suit jackets do have fashion cycles but whenever you wear this style, remember to keep the jacket fastened to avoid looking slovenly.

TROUSERS

Fit is of paramount importance. Stand straight and look in the mirror. Your trousers should hang in a clean line from the waistband whatever the silhouette or width—even a fit-and-flare trouser. If the fabric drapes from the side, clings to the thigh and then the calf, or cascades over your shoe tops (unless this is a specific design feature), the fit is incorrect. The fly may be zipped or buttoned, but should be smooth and not distorted. The seat should fit like fabric, not a second skin. The waistband must fit and should be neither so tight as to produce a roll of flesh above it nor so loose as to require support. If the fit is good everywhere else except at the waist, minor adjustments can be made. Good fit and comfort should combine, and the elements add up to a single statement.

MADE-TO-MEASURE SUITS

If you require any special areas of fit, it is wise to consider custom-made tailoring. Extra-long arms, very narrow shoulders, or a high rise (the length from crotch to waist) can all make life extremely difficult to buy ready-made suits. In the long term, the expenditure rewards the wearer, since an expert tailor can conceal figure faults, as the hang of each garment will be carefully calculated to compensate for these and create an illusion of perfection.

CARE OF THE SUIT

Having spent a great deal of time, effort, and money on a suit, care and maintenance are paramount. Your first purchase for the care of suits should be hangers. Wooden hangers with enough width to support the shoulders and a round, solid trouser bar that prevents creases forming are ideal. Don't cram suits into the wardrobe; a suit bag will trap some air within, thus preventing suits from being crushed. When you take off the suit remove all clutter from the pockets. This should never include anything bulky; pockets stuffed with such items not only spoil the line of a suit, but also stretch the fabric and give a disheveled appearance. Give the jacket a shake and fold the trousers carefully, then hang near fresh air before putting away. The fibers in fabric have a built-in elasticity that will respond to fresh air blowing through them, keeping your suit smelling fresh and looking crisp. A good brush and sponging is often the answer to minor soiling and damage.

BASIC OFFICE WARDROBE

This is a suggested starting point to take you through the first three months of a new job.

WARDROBE IN THE COOL COLOR PALETTE

Gray/blue tweed Crombie coat with gray velvet trim
Mid-gray plain suit:: 3 button
Light gray self-striped transeasonal suit: 2 button
Gray/blue fine check suit
4 white shirts (2 with French cuffs)
4 ice blue shirts (2 with French cuffs)
2 pale striped shirts
2 pale checked/herringbone or textured shirts
3 plain silk ties
3 textured silk ties
3 striped ties
3 brocade/patterned ties
1 pair silver cufflinks
1 pair pewter/gunmetal cufflinks
1 pair black lace-up shoes
1 pair black short boots/slip-on shoes
1 black plain belt silver buckle
1 black textured belt silver buckle
16 pairs black socks
16 pairs underwear
I gray/lilac/blue scarf textured/patterned
1 classic gray cashmere scarf
Black leather briefcase
Black leather document case
Gray carry-all/sports bag

ANATOMY OF A SHIRT

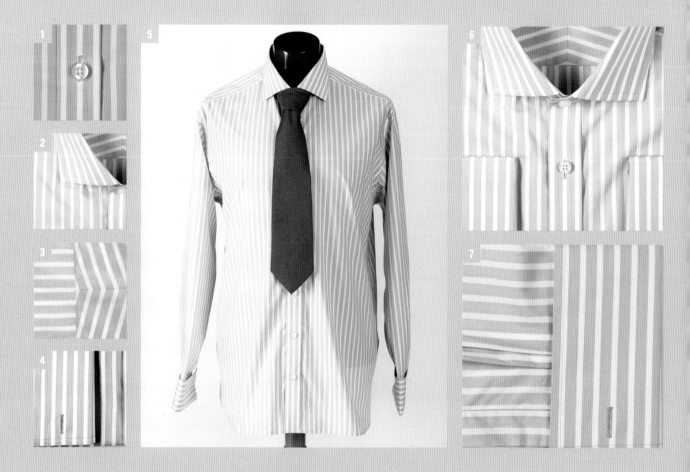

NAMING THE PARTS

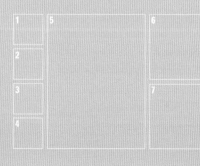

1 Small, neat buttons are classic and understated.

2 The cutaway collar requires a well-knotted tie.

3 Ease of movement is provided by the back yoke.

4 A french cuff ready for a top-quality cufflink.

5 Whatever the fashion of the day, a business shirt should be slim and well cut, neither voluminous nor skin tight.

6 Clean and unfussy lines characterize the perfect business shirt.

7 Pleats at the cuff allow for easy movement throughout the day.

Shirts come in a vast spectrum of colors, fabrics, and styles. Silhouettes can range from ultra-fitted to vastly oversized, and collars from collarless to huge Puritan collars. Buy shirts that match the rest of your wardrobe and the life you lead, and that combine in harmony of silhouette with the shapes that flatter your build.

SHIRT BASICS

FIT & SHAPE The construction of a shirt underpins the quality and the comfort. Too big a shirt, where the collar is loose when buttoned and the fabric of the body bulks up under your jacket, is obviously a mistake, but so are tight buttons straining across the chest and stomach, or a collar you cannot fasten under your tie; this is unflattering and uncomfortable and looks unkempt. Measure your neck and buy the correct size, check sleeve length when there is an option, and check whether a shirt is loose-cut, slim-cut, or fitted. Take time to ensure that the tails (which may be either curved or cut straight across) of the shirt are neither so long as to create a roll inside your trousers, nor so short they refuse to stay inside your waistband. Make sure that there is a yoke cut across the back of the shirt to allow for greater ease of movement. Try shirts on; don't assume they will fit. If you discover that certain makes work for you, return to them and buy with confidence. If you have shirts made to measure, all these problems are solved, but even then you may wish to purchase some ready-made items and work to discover the shirt maker who suits you best in fit and fabric.

THE STAND This is the height of the fabric supporting the collar, and it may vary from just a neat fold-over to the high, exaggerated Regency style. Obviously the shorter your neck the shorter the collars stand should be, and if you have a thick neck you should also avoid high collars.

Tip Keep your shirts stored in groups by color and purpose: hang the white city shirts separate from the weekend shirts. Put evening shirts and heavy winter or country shirts in their own sections. This will save you time in the long run.

THE SPREAD This is the collar itself, which may be made in one with the stand and is softer with a wide triangle silhouette at the front, or separate and attached to the stand with strong points almost meeting at the center. The spread width also affects the size of knot to be accommodated by the tie.

BUTTON-DOWN A style associated with preppy and more casual styles, the collar features two buttonholes at the end of the collar points to button onto the body of the shirt. Keep in mind that a crumpled, half-fastened collar looks disheveled, not casual.

TAB COLLAR A collar with an attached button tab to wear under the tie knot, forcing it forward.

ETON COLLAR A shirt collar with both a high stand and a rounded corner. This collar was popular in the Sixties in a soft version, as opposed to the correct version, which is highly starched and still worn by schoolboys at the prestigious Eton College, after which it is named.

CUFFS

FRENCH CUFFS The best option for a distinguished =business look, as well as for special occasion dressing, the French cuff is a classic for the well-turned-out gentleman, but it can also be a style statement on a weekend shirt in color or print. Remember that French cuffs can always be folded back for ease, since the weight of the extra fabric holds them successfully in place.

BUTTON CUFFS Also known as barrel cuffs, these may have one or two buttons to allow movement. Again, if work demands it, they may be folded back. Note that some cuffs have a double function for those who cannot make a decision.

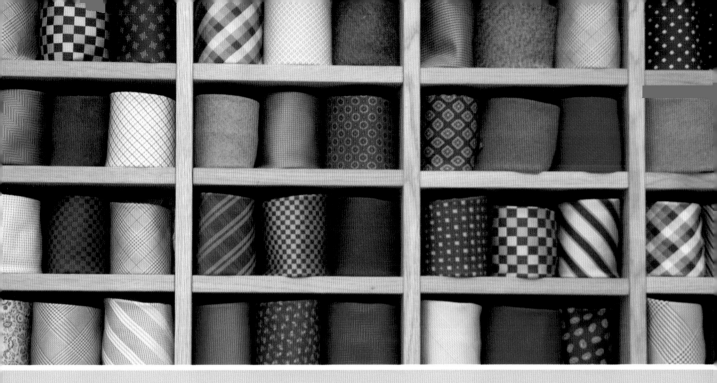

TIES

As early as the seventeenth and eighteenth centuries, cravats, scarves, and other neckwear were important elements of the sartorial style of a gentleman. Through Regency and Victorian times, neckwear continued to evolve and reflect fashion through knots, bows, and folds with length and width varying tremendously over the decades. However, the tie in a form recognizable today had appeared by the turn of the twentieth century and its evolution was completed in 1924 when Jesse Langsdorf, an American tailor, cut a tie on the cross grain of the fabric.

The width, length, and fabric of the tie may still reflect fashion's whims, and fluctuate in proportion to the current silhouette, but the tie is now established as a statement accessory to complete a look. It is a signal of status and attitude for many men: what clubs they belong to, what they consider appropriate for the occasion, and who supplies the tie. The tie is one of the few items of which a gentleman wearing one would ever discuss his maker, since the world's top menswear designers and suppliers make ties of outstanding quality.

CONSTRUCTION

The tie should be cut on the bias, meaning the straight threads run diagonally, not up and down. The tipping or lining should extend well up into the body of the tie. Check the weight of the tie by folding it around as if to tie it. If the knot looks unsatisfactory it shows poor construction. The details of the construction of the tie include hand-stitched bars inside to hold the fabric in place, a soft interlining, and enough ease in the sewing of the tie to allow stretch when being tied.

FABRIC

Silk is the usual fabric for a tie, whatever the fashionable style may be, but the silk itself can vary hugely. Self-color is when the fabric is either one flat color or tones of the same shade in the weave. Brocade is woven into a raised pattern, again in shades of one color, or fancy brocade when a jewel-like richness is added to the tapestry weave of the brocade with added colors. Brocades may be geometric, floral, traditional, or abstract in pattern. Foulard or conversational ties consist of small scattered patterns and paisley, which is based on Cashmere shawl patterns. There are prints that range from rustic and equestrian motifs to heraldic shields and florals. Club, school, or regimental stripes show the colors of the establishment to which you belong; these stripes generally, since the tie is cut on the cross, run diagonally. The stripes may be wide, narrow, or grouped, but should be woven into the fabric, not printed.

OCCASION

Town or country, formal or informal, fashion statement or classic, there are a dozen occasions to wear appropriate ties. Country ties may be knitted, wool, or wool and silk; the tie suitable for dinner at a fashionable restaurant in town would be inappropriate at a meeting with the board of directors; the tie for drinks at a club would not be suitable for the opening of an exhibition at an avant-garde art gallery. Not only do you need a selection of ties, but also you need to consider where and when they might be worn. Women will generally take an interest in a gentleman's tie, so their advice can be sought if you are uncertain.

CARE

Ties should last through several seasons and, since good quality ties are not cheap, should be looked after with care. Store ties either neatly rolled, with sufficient room to prevent creases, or hung on a rail or bar. Keep your ties in color groups and, if possible, style groups as well. Again, this makes selecting a tie a smooth business rather than a scramble for the nearest tie. Once a tie is old and tired, throw it out. Nothing looks worse than an outdated, dirty, stained, or badly knotted tie.

TYING A TIE

FOCUS ON THE FACE MEANS THAT NECKWEAR IS ALWAYS PROMINENT, SO REMEMBER, PRACTICE MAKES PERFECT—THE PERFECTLY TIED TIE IS A THING OF BEAUTY AND A SARTORIAL STATEMENT.

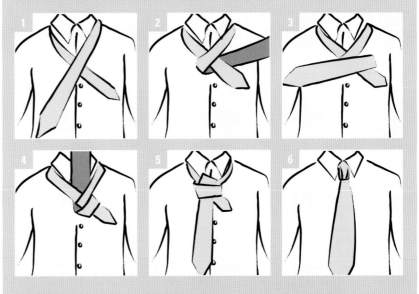

1. First fold across with the wide end on top.
2. Fold the wide end under.
3. Then wrap the wide end across the top.
4. Now bring through the neck loop.
5. Take the wide end through the loop.
6. Gently tighten the knot to fit.

COATS

A good coat is neither an impulse buy nor a fashion whim, so it is important to make your purchase in relation to your lifestyle and how often it will be worn.

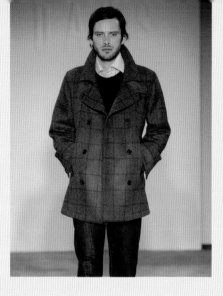

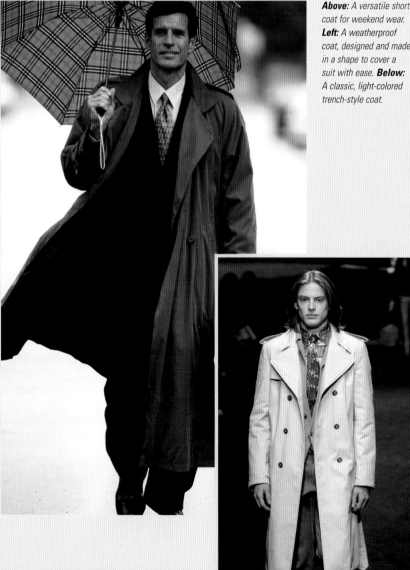

Above: A versatile short coat for weekend wear.
Left: A weatherproof coat, designed and made in a shape to cover a suit with ease. Below: A classic, light-colored trench-style coat.

TYPES OF COAT

You need to analyze the purposes for which you require coats before you purchase. If winters are severe where you live, or business trips take you to different locations and climates, it may be wise to consider two or three coat options.

TOWN COAT This should be a coat suitable for business and also classic enough to work with dinner suits and formal wear.

COUNTRY COAT The design and style should be easy in shape to wear over relaxed clothing on cool days, as well as when cold weather requires extra layers to be worn.

WEATHERPROOF COAT This may be based on a parka style, but is suitable for weekends both in town and the country. The coat will be made in a windproof and waterproof fabric, possibly lightweight and functional in design, and perhaps with multiple pocket detail.

Tip An excellent quality coat may be worth having re-lined if the lining has become worn or threadbare.

SHORT COAT This style was once called a car coat, since it was created to have less bulk when driving. Short coats are especially suitable for spring and fall when a heavy coat is not required. They often come in brushed fabrics and may also have an optional zip-out lining. Optional linings feature in a fair number of styles and are a marvelous idea if you can envision yourself zipping or buttoning them in and out; if not, leave them on the rack in the shop—they are not for you.

Tip Always hang a heavy coat on a good strong hanger to support the shape and fabric.

WINTER COAT This may be down-filled or parka-style, or it may be in a technical fabric, but the key here is that the coat is for extreme cold not just for a colder day. This type of coat may not get worn as often as others in your wardrobe, so it is wise to stay classic in design so that when it is worn it is timeless in style.

Right: A soft, neutral-colored Crombie coat, which will move from formal to casual.

TRENCH COAT The British classic is a coat with military styling including loops on the shoulders and a double yoke at the back; it is cut fairly loose and then belted. The classic trench always comes in shades of sand, beige, or taupe. The lining may be decorative in plaid or in a brushed fabric for warmth. The trench shape also comes as a classic belted winter coat in wool or wool and cashmere fabrics. Because the trench is belted, it is advisable to check if you have a waistline, since without one you will look like a badly tied parcel.

CARE Coats should be looked after carefully during their wearing time. Place them on a hanger and store them away, since throwing a coat over the back of a chair or hanging it on a hook will cause it to quickly lose its shape. Out of season, a storage bag with moth prevention inside will mean that when you next need the coat it will be in good condition. Give the coat a good brushing before storing and check for loose buttons or any needed repairs.

COATS

49

FOOTWEAR

The quality of a great pair of shoes is craftsmanship allied with practicality. The combination of beautiful leather, immaculate construction, and simple lines creates something from which you can derive endless pleasure. Cheap shoes cause pain and have little longevity, costing you more in the long run.

FIT

The form on which a shoe is created is called the last. If you discover a specific make of shoe that fits you well, it is because the last corresponds more closely to the shape of your foot than that of other makers. If you are able to have shoes made to measure, the last will be prepared to exactly replicate your foot and thus enable you to order without further fittings. The other matter to note with fit is that rarely are our feet a perfect pair; indeed, some people's feet differ dramatically. For this reason, it is important to always try both shoes on before purchasing.

Men's shoes come in an edited range of options, but the variety comes with not only the style but the weight; the heavier the task, the heavier the construction from leather to sole.

LACE-UP Shoes or boots with laces that tie at the front. The number of holes to thread the laces through can be from four upward, depending on the cut of the shoe or boot.

SLIP-ON These are shoes or boots that are simply pulled onto the foot. They may have an elastic insertion incorporated within the design for both fit and ease of wearing.

BOOTS The cut of the boot may finish on the ankle or above and the boot may pull-on or lace-up.

SPORT SHOES Sneakers, tennis shoes, deck shoes, and so on are just some of the varieties that originate in specialized sports activities. Many of them are now both ubiquitous in their application and worn by many patently unfit and unsporting types.

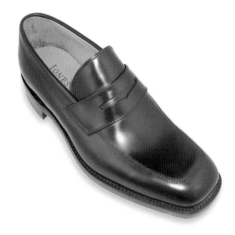

Above: Classic, top-quality shoes will last for a long time if well cared for. If shoes do not fit in the shop, do not buy them with the belief that they will stretch or just "need wearing." Of course, new shoes are much firmer in construction and fabric than old shoes, but shoes must fit in the first instance. Right: Socks and footwear should be in harmony; for example, a thicker sock for a boot and a rich colored sock with a polished brown brogue.

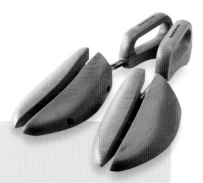

Right: *Cedar shoe trees keep your shoes looking and smelling better.*

SOCKS

Socks are often best purchased in bulk quantities and all old socks thrown out. Buy many of the same color and style and if odd ones appear they may be re-matched. Having a range of socks means choice and appropriate coordination in your top-to-toe look. Start with the classic plain or rib sock in black, navy, or dark brown as well as traditional discreet patterned socks, then introduce some colors for the weekend or the country. Heavy socks to wear with boots and athletic socks for sports activities can then be added, alongside socks suitable for wearing with sneakers. Fine or silk socks for evening and lightweight socks for high summer in town are other options. A wardrobe of socks will give you added polish and, since attention to detail shows your character, it is always a winner.

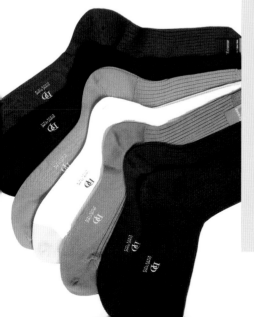

CARE OF FOOTWEAR
HOW TO CLEAN AND STORE YOUR SHOES

Polishing shoes both maintains and protects, along with communicating the impression of a man who takes time, trouble, and pride in his appearance. A properly stocked shoe-cleaning box is part of a well-turned-out gentleman's equipment. It should contain a range of polishes in blacks and browns, a selection of stiff brushes, and some soft cloths. For boots and specialized footwear, you may also keep grease, dubbing, and leather oil on hand. Always throw old or stale polish away. Use proper solid shoe polish and apply with a brush; leave for a brief period while the leather absorbs the polish. Then brush off the surplus and start to bring up a shine. Finish off with a soft cloth. Always pay particular attention to toes and heels and be sure to cover any scuff marks. Specialized and sport shoes require their own care and conservation, so read any instructions with the shoes as well as inquiring as to their care when purchasing sport shoes or sneakers. Some simply require washing, but others may require more elaborate cleaning.

Shoes should be stored with the toes stuffed or shoe trees inserted. Shoe bags are also useful, especially for frequent travelers. The key factor in shoe storage is to prevent shoes from becoming scratched and scuffed between wearing. Remember if shoes become wet to stuff them with newspaper while they dry, since leather stretches and if ≠left unattended the shape may distort. Shoes may be stored either in their boxes or on shelves. If stored in boxes it is a good idea to stick a picture of the shoes to the outside of the box for identification purposes.

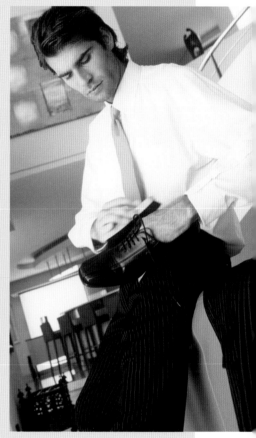

Tip *A long-handled shoehorn will prevent you from ruining the backs of your shoes by pressing, tugging, and distressing them as you put your shoes on.*

UNDERSHIRTS/T-SHIRTS

The classic undershirt and T-shirt have appeared in an extraordinary range of styles over the years. It seems that, though both garments are in theory classic, in practice we need to update them every season. This also means that it is important for a gentleman of style to reflect the current view of shape and detail. Both items have a noble history of practicality and are based in the manual labor roots of America. They are simple pieces with great strength of character and, especially in cinema and fashion, have become iconic in their application to image.

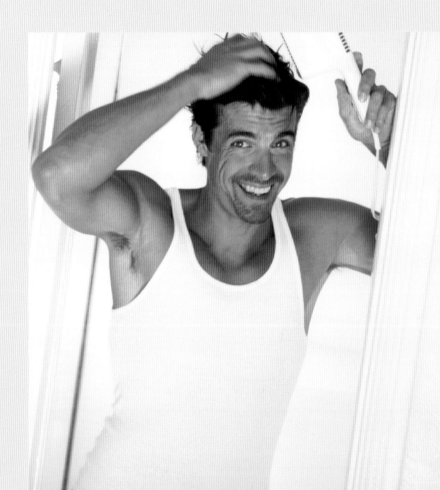

Left: *The athletic vest is for many men a preference over the T-shirt as either a sports item or underwear. Since it has no sleeves this garment can be cut and made tight to the body, and provide less bulk under a shirt.*

The undershirt and T-shirt are amazingly versatile: they can be worn as undergarments, as sleepwear tops, or as sport and vacationing items, and even with a tailored jacket. Since in all cases these items are worn next to the skin, they should be in white 100 percent cotton and top quality in finish. The stitching and ribs, or bands around the edges, should not be tight or chafe the wearer. These are also items that repeated laundering renders soft and comfortable, but bear in mind that although a ripped undergarment may look sexy in a magazine shoot, in real life you could just look shabby.

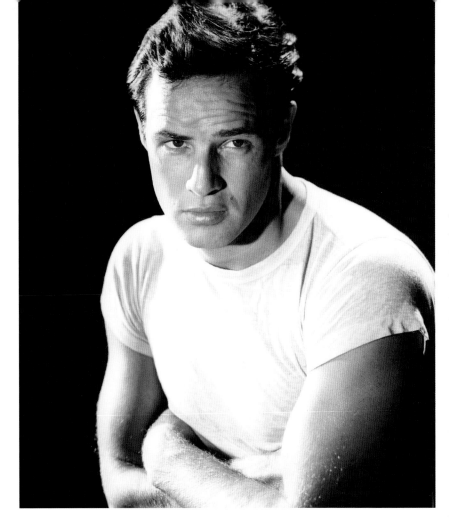

T-SHIRTS The white short-sleeved T-shirt is a simple classic item that has become a staple in the modern gentleman's wardrobe. However, the first thing that must be said is that it is not an easy garment to be worn solo. The high round neck and straight cut shape require a fit, trim torso, since the T-shirt emphasizes the contours of the body. Many men feel the T-shirt is a piece of clothing for everyone, but as you age and the weight piles on and the body droops, the T-shirt is unforgiving. Even when the T-shirt becomes an advertisement for a rock band, brand of beer, or a vacation destination, it is still not as ubiquitous in application as many men would like to believe.

A crisp white T-shirt under a summer jacket, showing at the neck of a sweater, or under a dark shirt is, however, a wonderful accent. Long-sleeved T-shirts have many of the same problems of figure emphasis as the classic T-shirt, but again are great as part of a layered look.

THE UNDERSHIRT The singlet, or undershirt, is a simple sleeveless undergarment designed originally for warmth and protection. The cut should be close to the body with a low neck and deep armholes. Designers will change this basic style over the seasons and years, but the classic undershirt is clean in line and unexaggerated. Among many variations, the most common are the racing back, which is cut away to provide more ease of movement, and the high-cut neck and armholes version, which moves the undershirt closer in style to a sleeveless T-shirt. Ribbed fabrics also provide variety in the look. The long-sleeved undershirt is based on Victorian underwear with a neat fine rib at the cuff and a neck opening with flat tape trim and two or three small buttons. This style is popular under sport shirts and weekend shirts for a rugged image. Often made in a heavier cotton jersey, the classic color for this item is ecru rather than white.

Tip *Printed, promotional, and designer T-shirts are subject to the whims and changes of fashionability. Be prepared to fold away beloved items when their day is over. An ill-advised band promotion T-shirt can make you a figure of ridicule.*

Tip *T-shirts change from year to year in subtle ways: V-neck, tightly ribbed fabric, boxy shape, and cap sleeves are all design elements introduced over the seasons, so be aware of these changes in style.*

boxer shorts, briefs, thongs, tangas & pouches, athletic supports & jock straps

UNDERWEAR

After bathing and before getting dressed, underwear is the first item of clothing a gentleman requires. The most intimate of apparel, underwear may not always be visible, but to the wearer, the comfort factor is paramount. Quality, fit, and style are the three key factors for purchase in all areas of clothing, but in underwear they are vital to your well-being throughout the day. You will also need to consider whether your life includes occasions, such as gym or other sport activities, when your underwear is on display, thereby making a visible style statement.

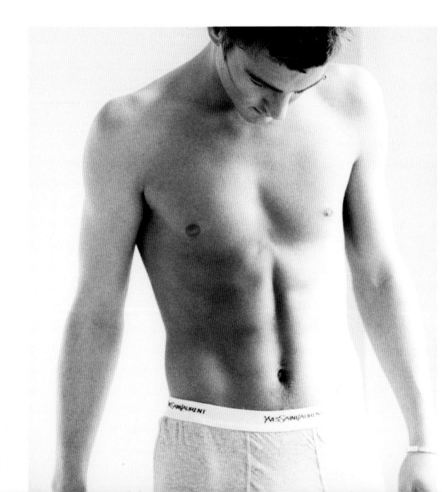

Underwear comes in a variety of colors and patterns; these are to be avoided. Buy underwear in a color that will complement your clothing and always have a stock of plain white. Plain white underwear launders well and looks fresh for anyone observing it, also during the summer it works well under light-colored clothing. Black underwear is also practical under dark suitings and jeans if there's a danger of dark dye colors being transferred. Fancy colors, patterns, and trimmings detract from the function of underwear—having a motley selection of styles, underwear becomes an unnecessary time-wasting decision in your life.

Tip The selection of style and fit of underwear will be dictated as much by personal preference and trial and error, as it will be by fashion; the choice is yours.

BASIC DRESSING

54

CLASSIC BOXER SHORTS So named since they are based on the style of shorts worn by boxers. Easy-fit leg shape with a firm elasticized waistband is the usual style. The classic boxer short has either an open or buttoned fly front, although some styles have no front opening. Cotton is generally the best fabric for this style, and the one most often used by manufacturers. Since cotton takes both color and print successfully, the options are virtually limitless. Novelty boxer short prints of animals or mottos may be contrasted with classic dark club-style stripes; perhaps neon print motifs can be seen next to discreet patterns; there is an overwhelming selection to choose from.

Tip Perhaps the best advice is the old adage, "If you were hit by a bus and rushed to the hospital, would you be ashamed of your underwear?"

JERSEY BOXER SHORTS This is a development from the woven style above, still with a longer leg and an elastic waist, but with many more variations in fit and shaping. Many of the jersey fabrics contain elasticized yarn, providing a closer fit and more support, and when this is combined with contour seams, it creates underwear that has a sport and streamlined feel. There are continued developments within this area of underwear with seamless and combination fabric structures and designs.

BRIEFS Briefs are cut in a simple shape, much like a classic swimming suit, that is cut to fit from waist to hip bone. Briefs may or may not have a fly or opening depending on the general style and contour of the brief. Made either in plain cotton or with added stretch yarn, the brief is again cut close to the body contours. Today there are also hipster briefs, mini briefs, and bikinis, which are all smaller-cut variations on the classic brief.

THONGS, TANGAS, AND POUCHES Tiny support garments based on posing garments from competitive weight training and modeling, they provide minimal front support and little other coverage. Such underwear tends to come either in basic sports fabrics or in luxury and decorative fabrics such as velvet or leopard skin print.

ATHLETIC SUPPORTS AND JOCK STRAPS The classic jockstrap provides a support cup with strong elasticized straps across the back. Once confined to locker rooms, the jock strap is now an option in underwear and comes in colors ranging from black to red. The primary function of this and other athletic support underwear is to provide suitable practical support for men in active sports.

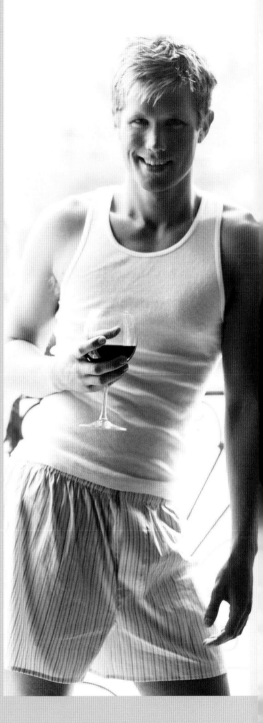

SLEEPWEAR

After the exertions of the day, retiring to bed should be a pleasurable finish. The choice of sleepwear and the items that accompany it can help you unwind as well as prepare for sleep.

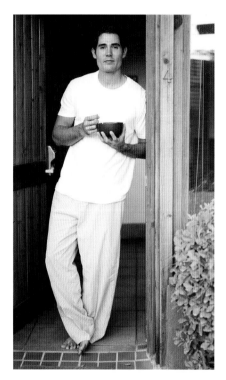

PAJAMAS The traditional choice for a gentleman is pajamas. A simply cut shirt with easy straight sleeves and a button front is teamed with straight legged trousers with an elasticized or drawstring waist. The truly classic fabric is cotton with a rich dark club stripe in shades of claret, navy, or bottle green. It is also possible to purchase pajamas with shorts for summer or tropical climates.

Tip Perhaps the most important factor to consider in sleepwear is the way the fabric feels against your skin, since your sleep experience should be one of ultimate comfort.

PAJAMA PANTS For many men, the bottom half of the traditional pajama is the only part they wish to purchase, perhaps worn with a T-shirt. Many designers now produce this style of trousers, which combines the softness of a pajama with the sportiness of a track pant. In either cotton or jersey, these trousers are generally in muted colors and classic plaid, and are also ideal as at-home wear.

T-SHIRT SETS A simple T-shirt and shorts made in the same fabric or color is a newer alternative to classic pajamas.

NIGHTSHIRTS Although in many ways the most old-fashioned, since they are based on the style of nightwear going back centuries, the idea of one simple oversized shirt-style piece still appeals to many men.

DRESSING GOWNS & ROBES There are two basic types of dressing gown: the classic shawl-collared tie-belt wraparound style and the oversized variety with either a huge collar or hood attached. The classic styles are in soft cotton for warmer weather made to match pajamas or pajama trousers. Winter dressing gowns come in warm, brushed, and comfortable fabrics. The second style is designed to be made in terry cloth since it is often worn over nothing. The terry style is increasingly popular and preferred by hotels that wish to make their guests feel as though they are wallowing in luxury. If you do purchase a huge terry bathrobe, make certain it remains spotlessly clean; food stains on any clothing are unattractive; on a dressing gown stains are simply slovenly. Also avoid turning your dressing gown or robe into some kind of comfort blanket that you retreat into at the first opportunity.

Tip Your choice of bedding will also influence your choice of sleepwear. Some men prefer light attire with heavy blankets and vice versa.

Right: Style doesn't stop after you undress. Robes and sleepwear should still spell class.

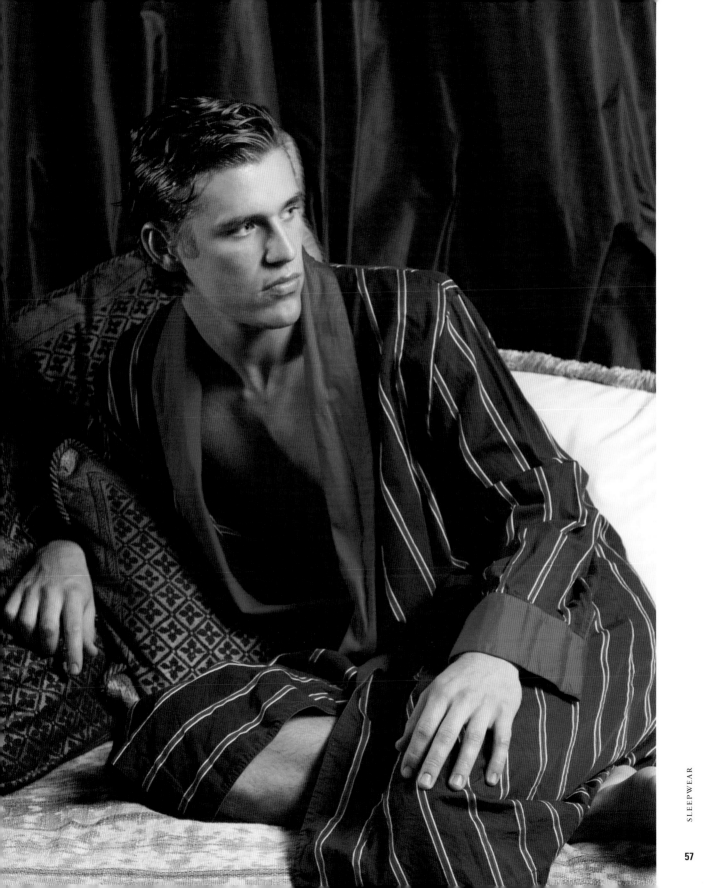

CARE & ORGANIZATION

There is little point in taking time and trouble to buy and wear clothes if they are neither cared for nor properly stored. Opening the doors to a well-managed closet should be like seeing one's well-stocked wine cellar—a source of pride and pleasure.

WARDROBE CARE KIT

Robust hangers

Suit bags

Shoe trees

Shoe bags

Shoe storage boxes/shelves

Belt hanger

Tie hanger

Sock and underwear drawer

Laundry bags—dark color/light color, wash and dry/wash and iron

Clothes brush

Lint brush

Sewing kit with white, black, and navy thread

Shoe box with polish, brushes, cloths

Steam iron

Ironing board

Trouser press (If you have room; best concealed in a closet)

(Note—Belts and ties may be stored rolled up in a drawer if space dictates)

THE CLOSET

Space may dictate the size of your closet, but this cannot be used as an excuse not to be organized and careful with your clothes. If space is at a premium, you should take even greater care to insure that your clothes are well cared-for in every way. Things to consider could include storing your vacation clothes in a suitcase or on a top shelf and using other available storage space to the best advantage; for example, storing underwear and socks in the bathroom or shoes under the bed in trays. In fact all organizational aids make life easier, including shoe racks, tie hangers, belt hooks, and storage organizers in general. The gentleman's closet should be arranged to conserve his purchases and to eliminate unnecessary wasted time locating items or fussing over clothing combinations. To help making choices easier, keep clothes sorted into formal or casual where possible, and also keep color coordinated.

Tip *Putting it all together should be based on knowing, first, what is in your wardrobe, and second, where and how to locate it.*

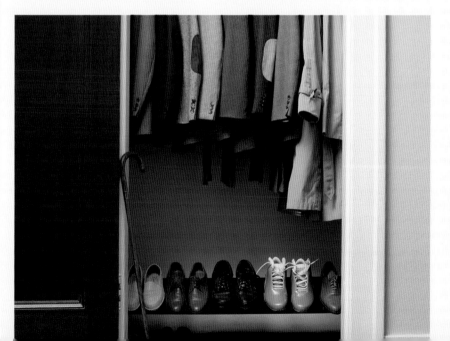

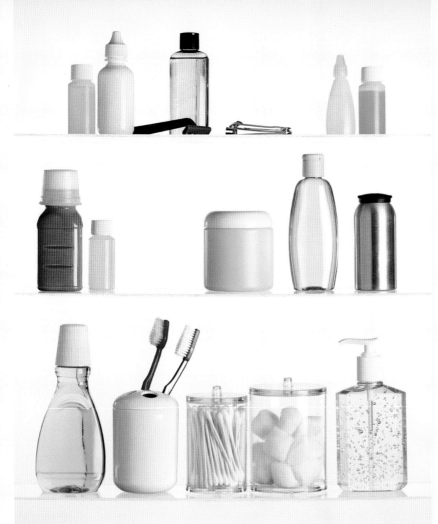

BATHROOM ESSENTIALS

Facial scrub or cleanser

Razors

Blades

(Shaving brush)

Shaving gel or soap

Moisturizer

Eye cream/neck cream/other

specialized moisturizer

Treatment mask or cream.

Tweezers

Small sharp scissors

Manicure kit

Pedicure kit

(Beard trimmer)

(Hair clippers)

Shampoo

Conditioner

Hair styling gel or cream

Toothbrush

Toothpaste

Specialized dental floss

Lip balm

Deodorant

Body moisturizer

Body scrub

Cotton swabs

Fragrance

THE BATHROOM

Good organization should also be applied to your grooming aids, from toothbrush to nail clippers. This avoids the disaster of discovering that you have run out of things, and also saves time in your daily work routine since everything is on hand. Never put away containers that have run out, and keep cabinets and drawers in your bathroom spotless. Replace nail clippers, tweezers, razors, and so on at regular intervals; do not wait until they no longer function properly. Spare shaving gel, toothpaste, deodorant, and other products stored ready for use prevents panic buying.

Specialized medicines and treatments for any conditions should be kept separate since organization and care in regard to these details ensures the smooth running of your daily routine and life.

The purpose behind this entire organization is simply to make life more pleasant in every way by editing and planning. You have the choice with a well-organized wardrobe to either plan and lay out your clothes before retiring for the night or collect them in the morning, since, with everything in its place, the time devoted to coordinating your style should be minimal.

Tip *Changing your clothes extends their life as well as marking the different areas and activities in your life.*

Above left: *Keeping things organized not only looks pleasing, but saves time and frustration; you know when stocks are running low since you can clearly view the contents.*

CARE & ORGANIZATION

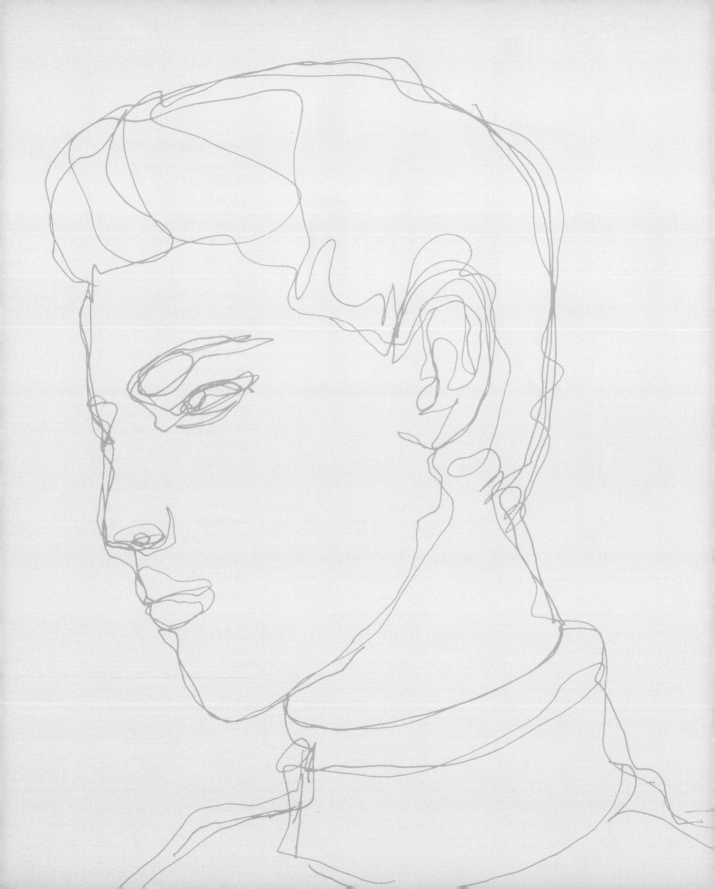

"Color inspires us and makes us feel, and makes us buy!"

LISA HERBERT, EXECUTIVE VICE PRESIDENT OF PANTONE, INC.

COLOR AND FABRIC

INTRODUCTION TO COLOR

It is a fact that which colors suit us and which colors we like may not be the same thing at all. You should select color for the improvements it can make to your appearance: color should enhance your natural hair and skin tones and flatter your contours. As extreme examples, imagine the result if a large, florid, red-haired man wore a red suit, or if a tall, pale, blond man wore a beige suit.

Color consultancy is a highly skilled, professional business and it can be money well spent to seek this kind of advice. However, be warned, not everyone who claims to be an analyst is actually qualified to do so.

GENERAL GUIDELINES

If you are trying to work out what color suits you, first consider your natural coloring (hair, eyes, and skin). Try some solid shades next to your skin; this will tell you very quickly what flatters you. Try, for example, a cool neutral (like a navy) and a warm neutral (say, brown) and see which works best. This shade will be the key to your color palette to build upon.

Tip *Always examine color in daylight as well as under shop lighting, since it may vary considerably.*

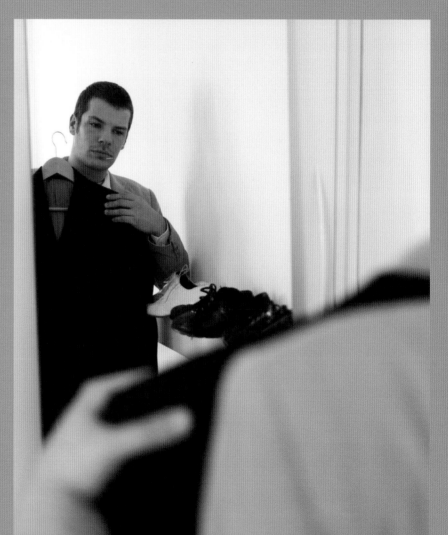

Right: *Check color in a mirror with good strong daylight, this will tell you the true depth and shade of the color.*

PALE If you have pale skin, soft blond hair, and your eyes are light blue, gray, or hazel, then you should try light shades that flatter and enhance your hair and skin (you'll need to wear as light a color as possible within the constraint of the occasion). Dark and strong color will drain and overpower you.

DARK If your skin is a strong tone from pale to dark, you have dark hair, and your eyes are dark, you should go for definite colors that emphasize your dramatic coloring. Pale colors will make you look washed out and soft neutral colors will make you disappear.

WARM If you have skin which goes from pale and freckled to warm and golden, hair which includes red (from true titian red to brown with a mix of red), and blue or green eyes, you should first check out the warm browns and neutrals (such as olive and terracottas), then add soft, warm accent shades. Pale tones can make you look washed out (particularly if they have blue undertones), and very strong color has the same effect.

COOL If your skin is pinkish in tone, your hair is silvery (from pale ash through to white), and your eyes are blue, gray, green, or light brown, you should go for clear colors that include greens and cool blues. Any blues are good on you, while other neutrals should be pink tinted.

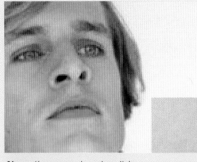

Above: Keep your color palette light.

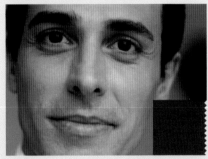

Above: Select your color palette for depth and strength.

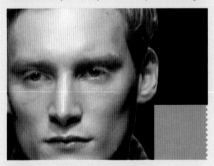

Above: Your key color palette is neutral and natural.

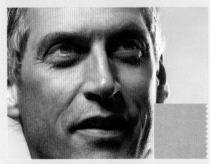

Above: A clear color palette is your best.

COLOR BALANCE

When choosing an outfit, whether city or country, formal or casual, the first thing to consider is the balance and proportion of color—what is the main color and what are the accents and highlights? For example, the wool fabric of a suit would be the major color for a business outfit; the shirt, shoes, tie, and accessories contribute to the color balance in varying proportions. Even if a color only appears in the cross check of the suit weave and in the enamel of your cufflinks, as an accent it makes the whole outfit more harmonious and alive.

Tip Colors you love but which don't suit you can be worked into your wardrobe in accessories and accents.

COLOR AND FABRIC

The fabric affects the quality and density of any color—and dictates how the color will wear and last. A deep shade in a cotton shirt that is regularly machine washed will fade and lose its density; a bright wool sweater that is carefully hand washed will retain its color for longer. Shine on a fabric's surface, like the silk of a tie, gives life to a color that in dull cotton twill looks flat. Synthetics often flatten color, while natural fibers such as silk, linen, and cotton avoid this; linen especially lends itself to rich summer colors and bright prints. Natural dyes in natural fibers fade gently, often to attractive tones of the original. Designers use this natural tendency as various washes and treatments for shirts, denims, and other natural fabrics fall in and out of fashion.

CLASSIC COLORS

The classic menswear colors are clearly defined and versatile. These colors are traditional and essential for every gentleman's wardrobe.

GRAYS This group takes us from black through the grays and finally to white. This is the monochrome palette and provides a shade to suit most colorings. Gray may have a slight color to it, from steely blue to a green tinge, but still qualifies as gray. Gray may also be soft and silvery or hard and dark. Black does not suit everybody top to toe at all times; as a gentleman ages and his skin begins to lose its tone, a dash of white next to the face provides a freshener. This palette provides a foundation for many men's wardrobes since it offers a versatile, yet timeless, color group to build upon.

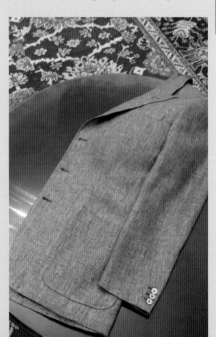

BLUE is a strong contender for the traditional menswear color of choice. It encompasses very dark navy, which replaces black for many men, and goes through to high summer blues. However, do not assume that you need blue in your wardrobe, as it does not flatter some men, although the stronger tones may be complementary when one is on vacation and tanned. Blue for summer and as an accent often contains hints of green, which can be surprisingly versatile with gray and brown.

Tip Carry small swatches of the key colors and fabrics in your wardrobe when shopping to make sure of color matches.

BROWNS The darkest shade of brown will replace black in the wardrobe for some men. Brown, like all colors, comes in a range of shades that have a tint, or a hint of other colors within them. Red, green, and yellow are among the colors found within tones of brown from deeper to pale. Warm and cool browns are also evident and should be checked for their suitability

Left: *Subtle shades of gray and blue are versatile suiting fabrics, and provide a background for accessory colors and patterns.*

against your skin, hair, and eye tone. Brown was traditionally never worn for business, and although this rule is more relaxed today, make sure the brown you choose does not look too informal. Brown can provide a great base for a surprisingly diverse and versatile number of colors from soft blue and lilac to geranium and turquoise.

NEUTRALS Neutrals are the soft colors that provide the basics of color play. They may be warm with a yellow tint or cool with a pink tint. Although seemingly safe, neutrals can be draining on hair, skin, and eye color. They can also become unflattering as skin ages and loses color, and they often need an accent to make them work. As a top-to-toe color look, neutrals work best in bright sunlight or with darker skin tones, or both. The neutrals are the colors above all others that require better fabrics to enhance them; cheap fabrics fail to encompass the subtlety and nuance that neutrals require to make them work. Nothing is worse than a kind of old oatmeal look to color and fabric.

Tip Don't forget, it is often your accessories that will complete your color style.

CLASSIC COLOR PALETTE
CHOOSING YOUR BASE COLORS

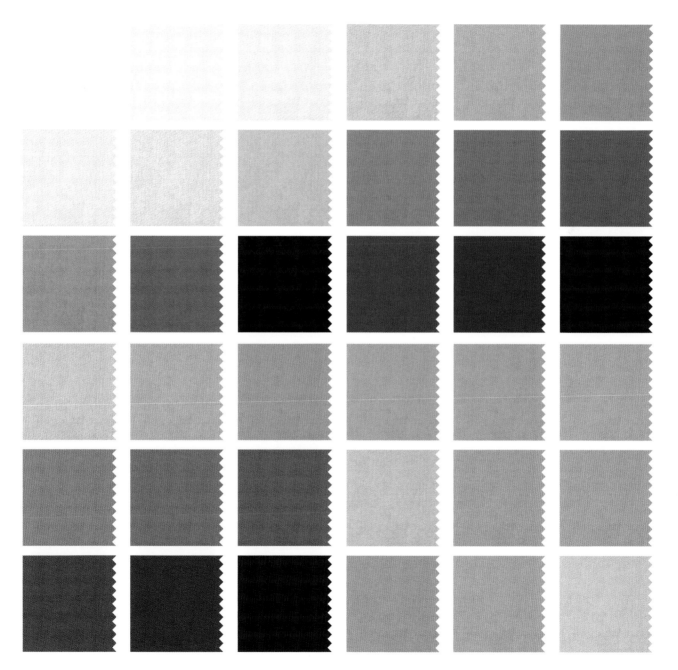

CLUB AND COUNTRY COLORS

These are the colors associated with any type of club, from the English gentlemen's club to sports teams. The colors are traditional in dense rich shades with brighter accents. They are suitable for both a silk tie and a striped polo shirt, and so transition readily from smart business to active sports style.

SPORTING COLORS Red, blue, and white, as well as green, orange, and yellow are the bright, highly visible colors appropriate for sports in one form or another. Sailing, baseball, skiing, or tennis: for whatever sport or sporting activity, including a great many spectator sports, the color palette is sharp and clean. These colors are also highly appropriate for the types of fabrics in this area of clothing, whether synthetic or natural.

NATURE'S COLORS This color palette takes its hues and inspiration from nature, whether fruit, flowers, or the seasons. These colors encompass the brighter shades as well as dense, saturated darker or mid-tone colors. Many of the colors in this group will be used primarily as accents for general menswear, but there are also times when these colors will be used boldly, such as for vacation wear, knitwear, and accessories. You must investigate these colors carefully to avoid looking either bland or unexciting. Playing color too safe is just as dangerous as overplaying it.

These colors also encompass the fashion shades, the dandy colors, and can be combined to make a country group of colors for each season from cool winter tones to warm summer shades, since the seasonal use of color in your workplace is an important statement.

Tip Light affects color. A tone or shade that looks good indoors in winter will look different outdoors in spring.

REDS Red can vary across an extraordinary range of shades with hints of blue, orange, or even pink shifting the tone, the depth, and the darkness of the color. There are purple tints to many reds and the use of red as an accent is helped by these deeper tones, which include the classic scarlet. The deep wine reds work with blue, gray, and some of the brown tones. They are also great next to club colors and rustic autumnal shades.

Tip Always try to select color with its general purpose in mind.

COMBINATIONS The colors listed and shown are by no means exhaustive, but they demonstrate the major parts of the gentleman's color palette. Color groupings such as tropical, autumnal, bohemian, or anything else the trends, press, and marketing representatives choose to call them, can generally be created through the colors listed.

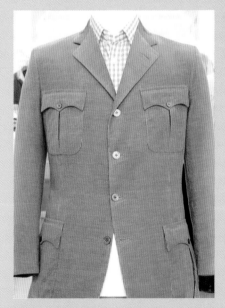

Above: *Country colors can be suprisingly vivid in town.*

CLUB, COUNTRY, AND RED COLOR PALETTES

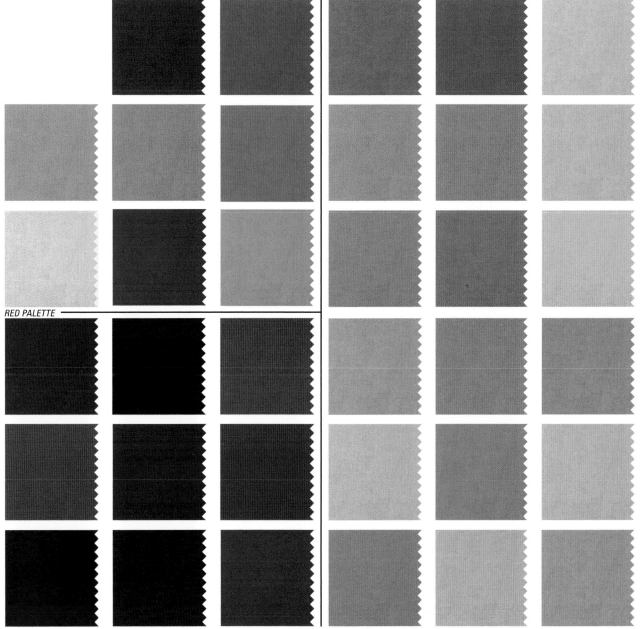

CLUB PALETTE

COUNTRY PALETTE

RED PALETTE

FABRIC

The most expensive fabric is not necessarily the best or the hardest wearing; a great deal has to do with the suitability of the fabric to the purpose of the garment. While luxury fabrics sound wonderful, the reason they are termed luxury is that they often have little functionality in their construction and may be almost fragile in their durability. The feel, weight, and texture of a fabric all add to its qualities; how a fabric stands up to washing, cleaning, and drying are other factors to be taken into account when looking at your wardrobe and the items you wish to purchase.

Ignore the fabric labels sewn into garments at your peril since they are often the maker's insurance policy. When buying a car, you check out all the details before purchase; you should do the same with your clothing—that way you do not get an unpleasant surprise. The percentages may also surprise you: just 5 percent of a secondary fiber may make a fabric tougher, more resilient, or simply easier to wear. Checking the fabric will also give you care guidelines so your purchases can be well—and correctly—maintained.

WOOL Wool is a natural fiber that takes dye and color well and is most notable for its warmth and, in heavier weights and knits, for its protective qualities against the elements. Wool is used for suits, knitwear, outerwear, coats, and accessories. Originally for cooler weather, wool is now available in a lightweight form for summer suits, as well as a wide range of wool-mix fabrics for many different purposes. Sheep are not the only animals that provide fiber for yarn. Some types of fleece yarns, including cashmere, alpaca, and pashmina, are spun from goat hair and the fleece of llamas.

COTTON Cotton is a naturally grown fiber that breathes with the wearer, hence its popularity for items worn next to the skin as well as for vacation and sports activities. As a bonus, it washes and launders well. Cotton comes as a woven fabric, as denim, and as jersey or knitted fabric. Stretch fibers are often added to cotton jersey and knits to help them keep their shape and support. Cotton is used for socks, T-shirts, underwear, jogging suits, shorts, trousers, shirts, and handkerchiefs. Cotton takes color and print well; it will, however, fade over time and print may wash out gradually.

LINEN Linen comes from flax, which is generally grown organically. It is a natural fiber, and as such it has certain inherent qualities. It takes natural and rustic color dyes best: ocher, rust, russet, burnt orange, bronze green, and deep teal. White, cream, and ecru linen is ideal for summer. Linen creases easily and, even when treated to be crease resistant, the fabric has a nonchalant, relaxed appeal with a soft crumpled surface. Unstructured jackets, pajama pants, soft baggy shirts, and easy shaped shorts are all favorite classic linen styles for high summer.

SILK A worm produces the silk yarn used to create this luxurious fabric. It has many forms: shantung—with a stiff surface suitable for waistcoats, lightweight dinner jackets, and accessories; brocade—again for waistcoats but especially for ties; and silk twill—woven with a fine diagonal rib, and the most common fabric for ties. Silk

CLASSIC FABRICS
WARDROBE ESSENTIALS

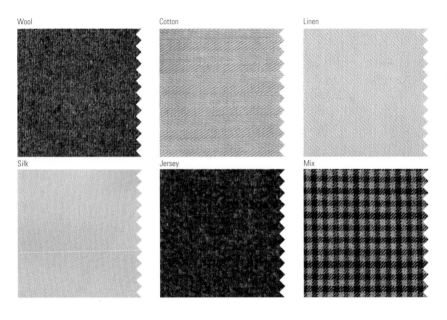

Wool　Cotton　Linen

Silk　Jersey　Mix

linen, silk, and cotton—can be woven, but the advances in technology now allow manufacturers to blend anything that achieves the correct weight of fabric. For this reason, it is wise to check out fabrics to be certain they are going to look good, wear well, and launder well.

MIXES Technology and experimentation mean that synthetics that were once less desirable for a variety of reasons can now be produced to simulate more luxurious fabrics, or blended with natural fibers to produce exciting and distinctive surface effects. Luxury fibers often require additions to stabilize their fragile qualities, so blends of fibers can often improve rather than cheapen a fabric.

SYNTHETICS Nylon, polyester, and Lycra are among the most common synthetic fibers. Yet there are many synthetic yarns and fibers, both mixed and used alone, within today's world of apparel. Originally many were created for one specific purpose, perhaps waterproof or easy drip-dry care. Now many of them are used in a multitude of ways and have moved away from the strictly practical and functional into the creative or even classic areas of your wardrobe. Synthetic fabrics have revolutionized sportswear from the simplest T-shirt to the newest sneakers. Again, it is important to read the label of many of these fabrics to understand their function and care.

added to other fabrics lends a touch of luxury and can even be used to create a fine knitted fabric. It is also used for sleepwear, loungewear, and some vacation wear. Silk takes all color without exception extremely well, hence the depth of color in ties.

JERSEY Jersey fabric is knitted and therefore has a certain amount of stretch and elasticity. The weight may vary from fine silk knits for undershirts and briefs to heavy wool jersey suitable for jackets and even coats. Since stretch is built into the construction, the fabric may also stretch when not required to do so, thus elasticized yarns are often added to stabilize the structure—as in socks. Cotton jersey is one of the most important fabrics in a

gentleman's wardrobe for underwear, T-shirts, and sweats. Sweat shirts and pants are made of cotton jersey of varying weights with a brushed backing. Cotton pique jersey has a textured pattern to it and is used for polo shirts and sportswear.

KNIT Knitwear demands its own set of rules—for details, see pages 104–105.

WOVEN A woven fabric is made up of the warp, the threads running up and down, and the weft, the threads running across, thus creating a weave. The classic woven fabric for a gentleman is made with a tight solid weave, but there are other looser weaves, such as linen weave, which are more open and transparent. All the natural fibers—cashmere, wool,

Tip *If you find stores that use fabrics you prefer and that wear well, don't hesitate to return. This isn't playing safe; this is common sense.*

SUIT FABRICS

Once you have discovered the silhouette and style of the suit that is appropriate to your figure, business, and pocket, there will be the fabric to consider. If you are small-framed and require neat uncluttered tailoring to make you look your best, then it follows naturally that discreet, quiet, and minimal patterns and weaves will further flatter you. Stripes, checks, and herringbones, classic though they all are for suits, can all come in a staggering array of sizes and colors.

CLOTH There is one simple infallible rule for choosing a suit fabric—feel it and squeeze it. If it feels rough and coarse to the touch, wherever it comes in contact with your skin it will itch and irritate. If the fabric fails to bounce back to flatness after twisting it into the palm of your hand, the fabric will crease and leave you looking disheveled and unkempt.

Suit fabrics are predominantly wool-based for all seasons, varying in their weight and weave from heavy for the coldest climes to lightweight for the tropics. The wool may also be blended with other fibers in varying proportions. Silk and wool, polyester and wool, and cashmere and wool, are all possible variations and appear in a wide range of qualities. The design firm of Armani has developed suit fabrics with superb surface effects, and the great Italian mills produce truly delectable fabric that explores and develops fiber combinations. Wool flannel has faded from the suit market

as it is difficult to make light enough for modern business wear and still retain the intrinsic quality of the fabric; however, it is still a great fabric for casual wear, especially in blazers.

Mohair suits were popular in the 1950s when it was created as we know it today. The best examples of this look are to be seen in photographs of the Rat Pack members. At various times it has been revived, as have alpaca and vicuna.

Tip Check out the fashion in men's style publications to see the most popular variations of classic fabrics for the season.

PATTERN Checks and stripes in suits should be subtle and flattering. Chalk stripe (large) and pin stripe (small) are the most classic stripes and can vary from soft tonal highlights widely spaced across the fabric to bold graphic white only set apart by a few inches. Always try a complete suit on

to gauge the effect on your particular body type when selecting a stripe and stand well back from the mirror to get the full impact of the stripe. Other stripes in suiting may introduce fine single thread accents of color, or shades of the main color; these features also apply to checks. Prince of Wales, dogtooth (small) and hounds tooth (large) are some of the checks which are to be found in suit fabrics and again the scale is wildly variable. Herringbone is the chevron-style pattern that for the casual look is bolder than in business attire, where the herringbone weave is often virtually invisible. Suit patterns and textures generally are understated and discreet to allow for many wearings which, with changes of shirt and tie, create the illusion of endless variations on a theme.

Tip Surface-effect weaves can look good close up, but may not work as a whole suit, so always be sure to try on before buying.

SUIT FABRICS

SUIT FABRICS ARE CHARACTERIZED BY THEIR DISCRETE PATTERNS AND PRACTICAL COLORS APPROPRIATE FOR BUSINESS.

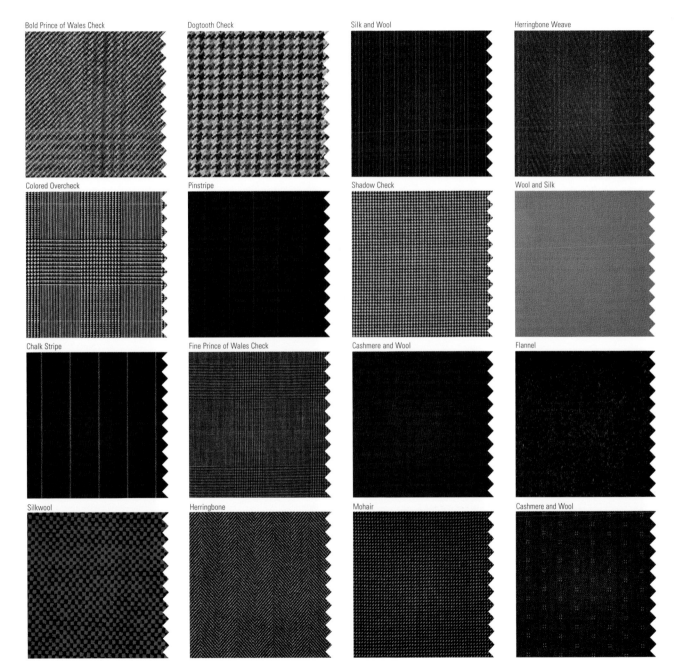

Bold Prince of Wales Check

Dogtooth Check

Silk and Wool

Herringbone Weave

Colored Overcheck

Pinstripe

Shadow Check

Wool and Silk

Chalk Stripe

Fine Prince of Wales Check

Cashmere and Wool

Flannel

Silkwool

Herringbone

Mohair

Cashmere and Wool

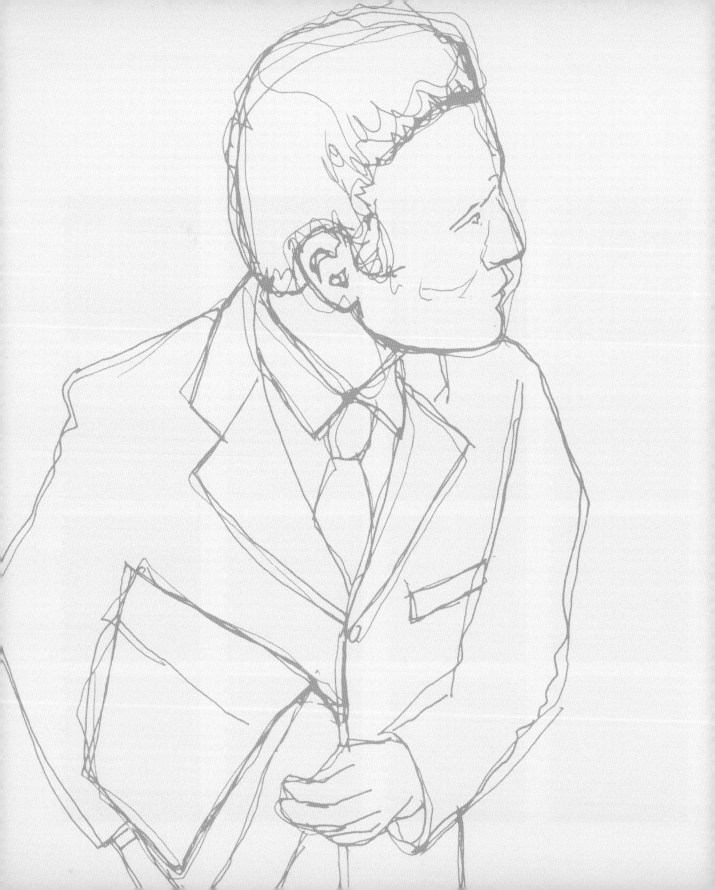

"The suit is … worn by men of all classes when a declaration of social position and polite behavior is demanded."

HARDY AMIES, SAVILE ROW TAILOR AND ROYAL DRESSMAKER TO THE QUEEN OF ENGLAND, ELIZABETH II

DRESSING FOR TOWN

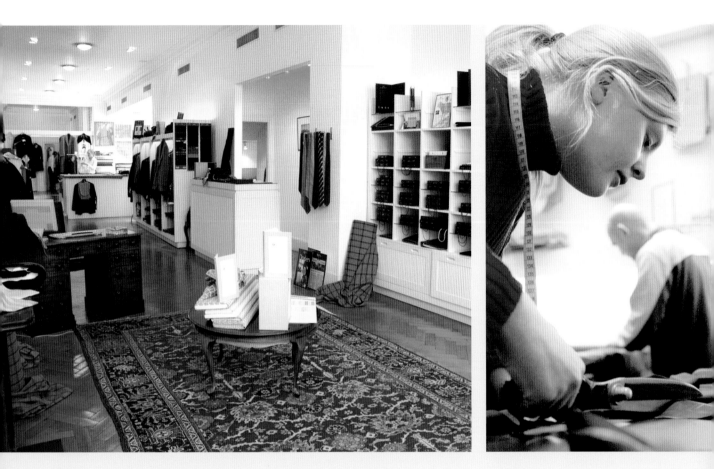

BUSINESS SUITS

A suit may speak volumes about its wearer, both good and bad, which is why, in formal business and professional situations, your choice of suit really does matter. The suit is a relatively modern invention, but as a tool for promotion, a weapon for boardroom coups, and a statement of success, it is unparalleled. Although "the suit" in one form or another has been a term for men's apparel since the late 1600s, the suit, as we recognize it in the form of matching jacket and trousers, only came into fashion in the late nineteenth century.

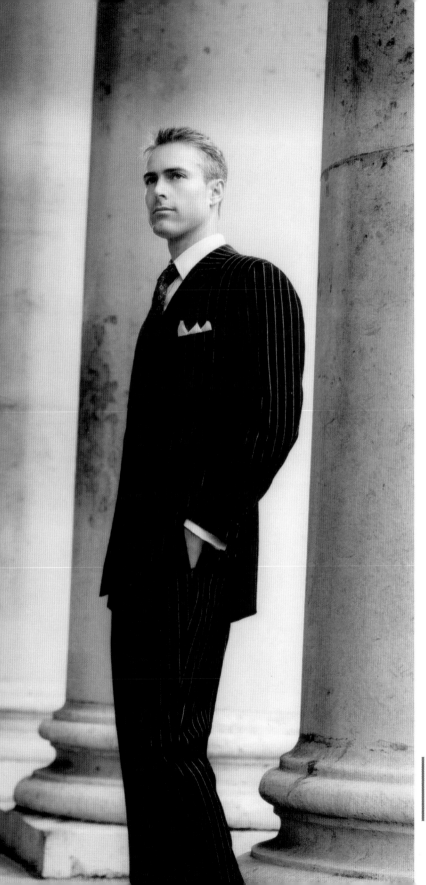

There are two options. Made-to-measure or tailored is the equivalent of women's haute couture in that each garment is made to fit the wearer and is totally exclusive to the individual client. The alternative is the off-the-rack or ready-to-wear garment, which may be purchased at any number of retail outlets, depending on price and quality level, and which comes in standard measurements. However, many first-class shops and stores do provide alteration services for hemming trousers, shortening sleeves, and other minor modifications.

Do not imagine that an ill-fitting off-the-rack suit can be made into a perfect fit by a few minor adjustments if the basic structure is all wrong; the suit will never fit properly and, each time you try it on, it will reproach you as a waste of money. Better to spend more time and money and be satisfied.

DESIGN OF THE BUSINESS SUIT

The aim of a well-dressed gentleman is for the proportions and silhouette of his tailoring to flatter his figure and display harmony and balance. Each element must be considered in the overall picture. Fabric, color, length, shoulder line, vents, pockets, cuffs, and collar are all changeable elements within the construction of a suit.

Tip When purchasing a suit, try to balance between repeat buying and impulse buying—in other words, consider what you already have and what you need.

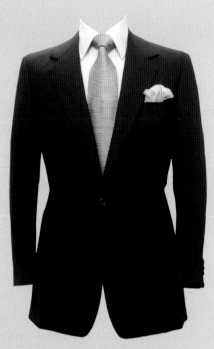

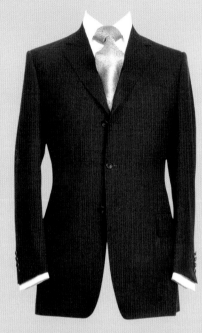

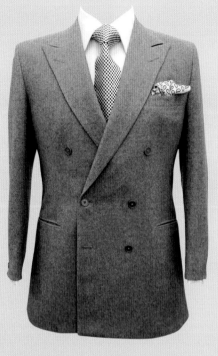

Above: *The single-breasted jacket with a lower buttoning creates a slim-shaped torso.*

Above: *A single-breasted, three-button jacket is flattering, the vertical emphasis is created by the clean center line. Avoid styles with high buttoning, this can exaggerate the chest and stomach.*

Above: *A double-breasted jacket emphasizes the waist and stomach, making it a bad choice for the larger man.*

In the last fifty years, the structure of the suit and the weight of fabric have relaxed dramatically. Rigid canvas interfacing, padding, and stitching combined with heavy wool and worsted fabric belong to an age before central heating and air conditioning. Lighter fabrics and softer fusing have given the suit a contemporary feel. Designers have worked with tailors and craftsmen to bring the construction of the suit into a modern version of a great classic. Formalwear and suits are seen as style statements that have been partially affected by the demise of dress-down days, which are now deemed less conducive to successful business and may

even decrease productivity in the workplace. This is reflected by the number of men, in entertainment and creative industries especially, who see the well-cut suit as a statement of serious intent and overall success in their specific sphere of activity.

Tip Never overdo color matching; it will look effete and contrived. Tie, socks, cufflinks, and handkerchief all bringing out the color of the shirt, which matches the tie, is a step too far.

Check up on fashion details in magazines and the press: Are turn-up collars back?

Should you go for two buttons or three? Are lapels getting wider? Should you choose single or double vents? A suit with style is often all in the details. Try the suit on. Notice that if you have a smaller frame it is safer and more flattering to stick to few and small details and subtle fabric designs. Let broad chalk stripes act to enlarge to your physique, but never be dwarfed by your suit.

Tip A suit purchased in haste, and with insufficient attention, will result in sartorial disaster.

BUSINESS SUIT PATTERNS AND COLORS

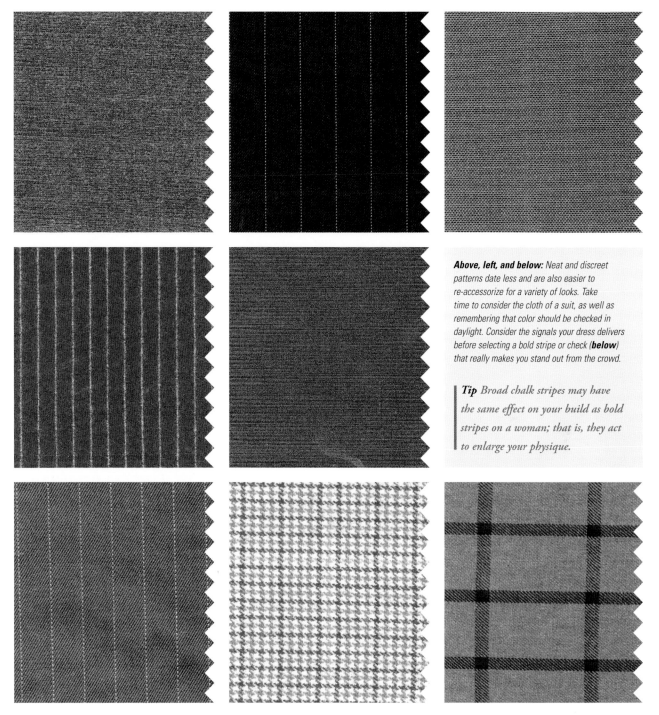

Above, left, and below: Neat and discreet patterns date less and are also easier to re-accessorize for a variety of looks. Take time to consider the cloth of a suit, as well as remembering that color should be checked in daylight. Consider the signals your dress delivers before selecting a bold stripe or check (**below**) that really makes you stand out from the crowd.

Tip Broad chalk stripes may have the same effect on your build as bold stripes on a woman; that is, they act to enlarge your physique.

SHIRT TAILORING

A beautifully made business shirt is an item to cherish and to wear with both pride and comfort. A cheap or inferior quality shirt may have many annoying elements—bad fit, rough collar, insecure buttons, and nasty fabric. During a long day at work, a shirt should retain its crispness and the collar and cuffs remain in pristine shape. Frayed cuffs and a pinched collar on a crumpled shirt do not inspire confidence in either your co-workers or management. Good shirts are money well invested in your wardrobe, since they have to stand up to a great deal of wear and tear and repeated laundering.

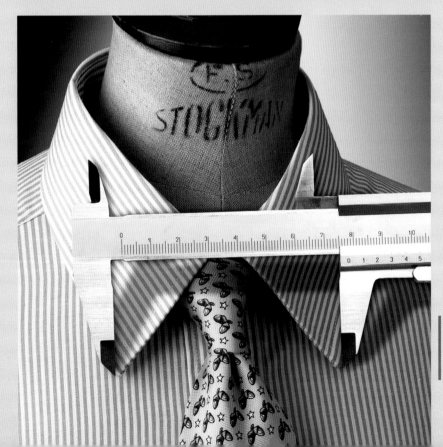

COLLAR STYLE Fashion often dictates seasonal collar fads, but while a gentleman may modify his style, ultimately he should select a spread of collar that suits his face shape, thickness and length of neck, and suit style and remain true to the overall concept. Remember that collars on shirts have two key elements and style factors to consider *(see Anatomy of a Shirt, p. 44)*. For a round face and a short, stout neck, the modified pointed collar with a shorter stand to it is more comfortable and flattering; conversely, for a long face and a long thin neck, one should look for a shirt collar with a deeper stand and wider spread.

Tip If a business shirt becomes tight, get rid of it; a tie pushed up to cover the fact that you are unable to button the collar of your shirt does not give a good impression.

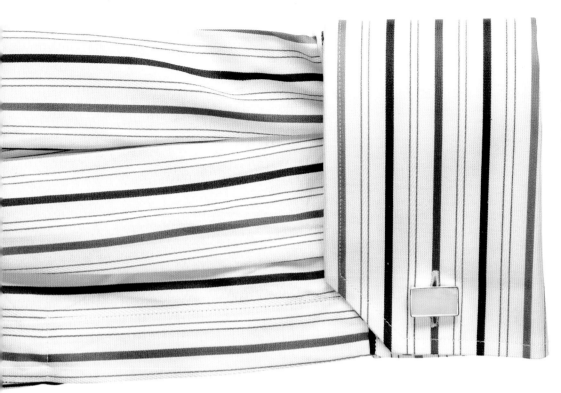

FRENCH CUFFS These are the best option for a distinguished and polished look. The double fold of fabric and the accompanying cufflinks make a statement of professionalism and quality. The cuff itself is an expression of luxury and quality since the double fabric is neither a necessity nor fashion; it is the true classic cuff style for business. The shaping of the cuff corners may be rounded or square and should be in harmony with the collar shaping. Cuffs should always be gently folded back for more demanding and physical work at the office to protect them from soiling; this gesture will also convey a willingness to "roll up your sleeves" and get on with work.

Tip Heavy designer motifs or fancy buttons have no place in a gentleman's business wardrobe.

If you are really averse to French cuffs, make certain that you buy shirts with a well-structured and crisp cuff. Check the quality of the buttons, which will be shown off in the same manner as cuff links. You may also select a design which features two buttons, one above the other, making a subtle design statement. This is not to be confused with the buttons side-by-side on a shirt cuff, which are intended for the tightening of the cuff.

In general, shirt buttons should be made of mother of pearl which has a discreet surface sheen and luster. Buttons should have four holes for attaching them to the shirt fabric and a neat rim or ridge around the edge. This is the classic shirt button and, although the buttons may be substitute resin, this is still the best option for business shirts.

SHIRT FABRICS

All shirts should be 100 percent cotton, since blended fabrics are often less absorbent and are liable to pill, and quickly lose their color. Fabrics that are too soft can look tired by midday at the office, so choose a fabric with a firm texture. This applies to weekend shirts in corduroy, brushed cotton, plaids, or even floral prints. The thread count should help with quality of cotton, but this is not always indicated, so go by touch. Synthetics can be useful for vacationing shirts, but check carefully for creasing and ease of cleaning; there is no point in buying a vacationing shirt that creases in the suitcase or cannot be washed and dried overnight on a hanger.

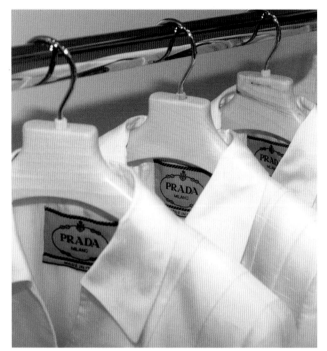

SHIRT FABRICS AND COLORS

For much of the time only a small part of a business shirt is visible, yet great importance is attached to having the correct shirt. In fact, the very emphasis on that small area of focus on the collar and cuffs, and how the color and fabric can flatter or detract, is what makes it such an important garment in a gentleman's wardrobe.

FABRIC

The choice of fabric is a major contributor to the comfort and style of the shirt. One hundred percent pure cotton is a natural fiber that breathes; it is also surprisingly resilient and practical since it stands up to hard wear and repeated laundering. The business shirt should be the best quality you can afford, and, since cutting-edge design plays a small role in your business wardrobe, purchasing classic shirts in top-quality fabrics on sale is a good option.

Tip Always consider the suit fabric your shirt fabric is to complement. There should be a subtle relationship of pattern and color either complementing or accenting the suit fabric to the shirt.

OXFORD CLOTH is not for businesswear and indeed self patterns in white-on-white can also look crumpled, even direct from the laundry. Discreet woven stripes in fine colors to be picked up in either the tie or suit are classic without being boring. Bold stripes, at present, belong at an 80s party unless you are certain you have the panache to bring them off. Very fine checks can be a good alternative, but do not go well with every fabric, thus you should beware of looking too casual with some checked patterns. Contrasting collar and cuffs, sharp white on either a striped or colored body, can look strong and snappy, but this is very much a style statement and only you will know if it is appropriate to your profession and personality.

COLOR

White is best. Why? In the workplace with often dark surroundings and also matte dark suits, an accent of white shows up as both crisp and efficient, as well as drawing attention to the face and hands when you are making statements and gestures in a conference. A crisp white French cuff with suitable cufflinks gives an impression of elegance and confidence. A beautifully knotted silk tie is shown at its best by a sharp white collar. White also prevents time wasted in coordinating your attire: a white shirt goes with everything.

Above: Even with very subtle variations in fabric, a shirt can be classic yet still make a style statement. The perfectly cut shirt in great fabric is a work of art to be conserved.

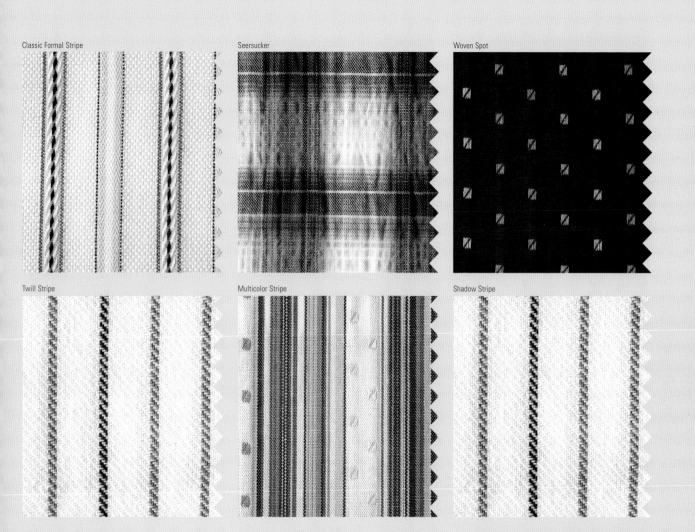

Classic Formal Stripe

Seersucker

Woven Spot

Twill Stripe

Multicolor Stripe

Shadow Stripe

IVORY AND CREAM These colors of shirts are difficult in that they frequently look off-white. It is better to go toward a more definite shade, such as buttermilk, so that your shirt doesn't appear dirty or graying. These colors add a touch of vintage elegance.

Above: *Shirt fabrics are surprisingly interesting. Take time to scrutinize and handle before purchasing.*

BLUE is the second color of choice for business. From strong sky blues to ice blues, there is a shade of blue to suit most complexions and styles. Again, the blue shirt is best in a plain classic fabric, perhaps with a touch of sheen to the surface. Pink, pale lavender, palest lemon, and other tinted colors can also provide a lift to the plain shirt, especially in spring when they bring a breath of freshness to the workplace.

BLACK SHIRTS and very dark colors have been in fashion in recent years, but they are specialized in their application for business use. Above all other considerations, the dark shades wash out very quickly after repeated laundering, thus looking poor and tired.

Tip *Old-fashioned though they may seem, sleeve bands really do work, especially if you want to keep cuffs pristine.*

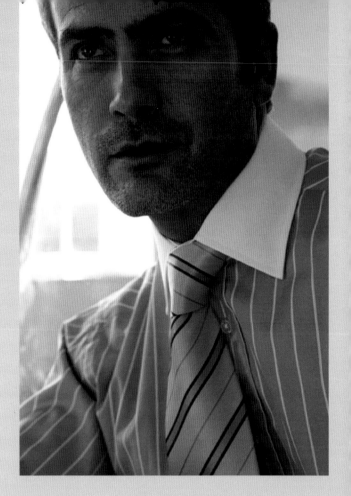

TIES

One of the most important statements a gentleman can make in the workplace is with his tie. Everyday office routines, board meetings, interviews or lunches with colleagues; each occasion requires thought as to the signals a tie might send out. When selecting a tie for the office, it is important to take into consideration the day-to-day routine of your working life, as well as social occasions that require a tie.

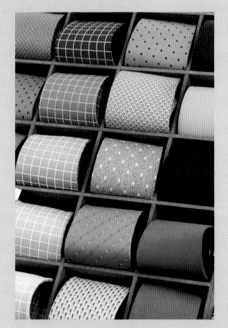

SHAPE As fashion and style move across the seasons, so the width and shape of the tie gradually evolves. Think of the straight, narrow ties of the late 50s and early 60s, or the kipper tie of Swinging London's 60s look, and you can see how style changes dramatically. Bear this in mind when purchasing a tie; your aim is to look stylish yet neither exaggerated in your dress nor a fashion victim.

KNOTS There are several classic knot options (*see Basics, p.47*), but the size of the knot is obviously affected by the width of the tie. Generally speaking, the knot should form a neat fold, then flare out. After you tie the knot, slip the under piece into the band on the back of the broad blade to keep it anchored. Never knot your tie so the slimmer end is hanging below the wider part.

Tip Always check that your collar is turned down all the way around, after knotting your tie.

FABRIC The key to purchasing a tie to be worn in business is to select a tie for daily use that is classic and versatile. You may then buy ties with a special occasion look to them: a tiny floral pattern for a spring or summer lunch in town, a graphic stripe for giving a presentation, a neo-classical brocade for meeting senior members of the board.

Left: *Every man prides himself on his tie collection, but make certain it reflects style as it changes over the years.*

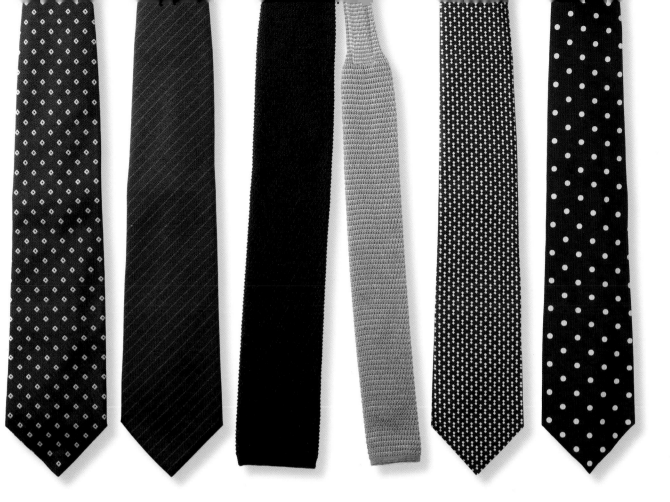

COLOR A tie that incorporates shades related to your suits should also be capable of being worn with a variety of clothing. When considering color, consider the occasion, the season, and the time of day. One example might be a winter afternoon meeting followed by drinks, a presentation, and then dinner; another might be a presentation on a spring morning, a sandwich at your desk, and a meeting in the afternoon. The first scenario would require a darker, richer, and more formal tie while the second would be suited to a low-key, softly colored tie in a micro pattern.

Tip *Think carefully, and take time before purchasing a tie and you may save yourself a great many sartorial faux pas.*

Above and right: *Bold or subtle, colorful or somber, selecting the appropriate tie is always a question for careful consideration.*

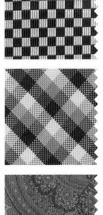
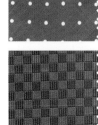

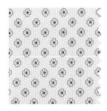
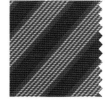
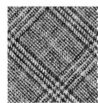

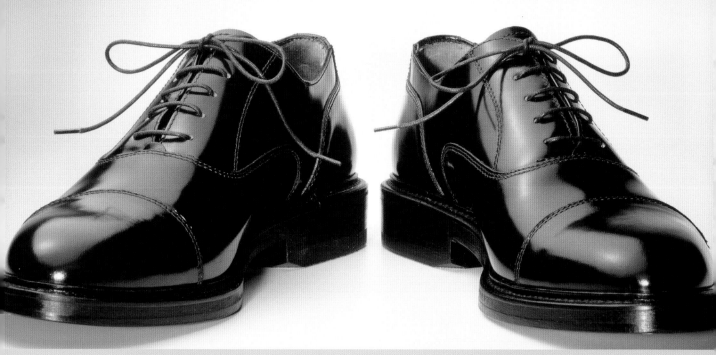

BUSINESS FOOTWEAR

Business shoes come in a wide range of styles but are defined by one key stylistic element: lack of fuss over elaborate design details or tricks. The perfect professional shoe is defined by both its initial quality and the high level of maintenance the wearer devotes to his footwear investment.

Bear in mind that in the past shoes have been passed down from father to son; this reflects the style of classic quality footwear for town. Fashion may dictate extremes of shape and decoration; the gentleman will rely on quality and timeless perfection in his choice of shoes.

QUALITY & COLOR

Your business shoes should only ever be noticed for their quality; they are not a fashion statement. If properly cared for (*see Basics, page 51*), well-made classic shoes should last many seasons and will never look out of place.

Classic for color is of course black, which will go with all dark suit shades. Black may also be worn in town with lighter spring suits and shades of gray. For a wardrobe with suit fabrics that contain an element of green or brown within them, a very dark brown shoe may be worn.

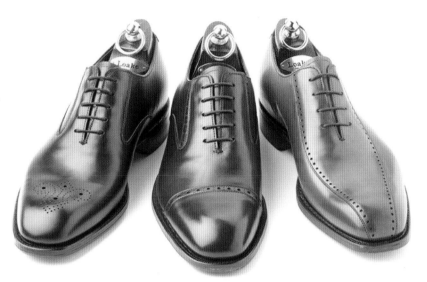

STYLE

THE CITY BROGUE The shape should be oval-toed and the style lace-up. The sole should be sufficiently stout for walking and repairs, but not heavy enough to resemble a workman's boot. The punching or brogue detail should be classic in form and the laces should be clean and neat, never old and knotted.

Tip *Rustic and lighter browns along with tan and earth-based colors are more suited to the country than for formal wear.*

THE CHELSEA BOOT A modern city style derived from a short riding boot. Once again it should be oval-toed with either neat elastic insertions or a fold-back strap and buckle, in plain metal, at the ankle.

THE LOAFER AND SLIP-ON Oval-toed and plainly cut is the style for the city. Elaborate or fussy details have no place in business. The shoe may be high-cut over the instep or with a neat strap in the classic style. Classic penny loafers can look too casual for formal business wear, but are a good business casual or weekend shoe, as are tasseled loafers.

Tip *For comfort and sartorial style, you should always buy the best shoes possible. The damage done to your feet by ill-fitting or cheap shoes is irreparable.*

Left and Right: *Even the most classic of shoes comes in a range of variations and subtle advances in style. Dark socks to match shoe tone are best for work; if you want to make a statement, go for a color that matches your shirt.*

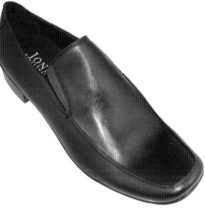

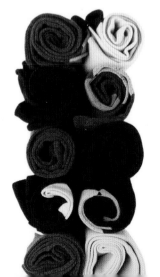

BUSINESS SOCKS

Socks worn with a business suit have but one purpose: to cover the foot, ankle, and calf. In Italy, city socks often seem extremely long, but at work a gentleman should be secure in the knowledge that his socks are long enough. The casual sock is not an item of clothing for making a statement. Socks must be closely toned to the suit, in an appropriate weight, and always spotlessly clean.

PLAIN SOCKS Micro-patterns and semi-plain, ribs, and self patterns give these socks character.

PATTERNED SOCKS Tone on tone pattern, fine dots or stripes, and the classic clock, which has a motif across the ankle.

COLORED SOCKS Deep tones that may pick up on a check or stripe in your suit or shirt are best. Avoid very strong colors, such as red.

BUSINESS COATS

Any coat in a gentleman's wardrobe should be a practical and long-lasting item. Fashion may, however, influence the silhouette, construction, and style of overcoat over several seasons. Under no circumstances, though, must fashion lead you to purchase a purely decorative, impractical, and one-season-wonder coat. A coat of quality and function is an investment piece that should be classic enough to be worn over several winters, yet with key elements of style, rather than pure fashion, carefully analyzed.

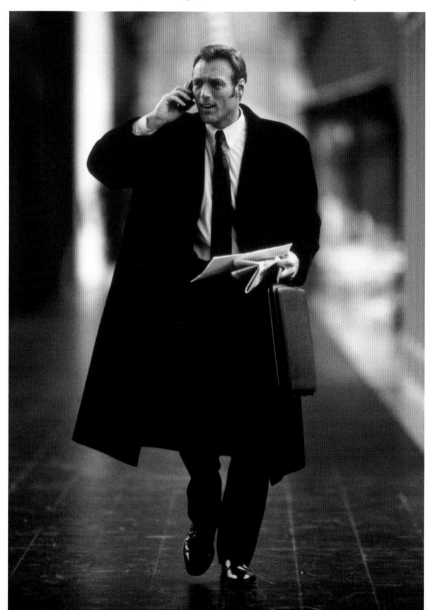

CLASSIC OVERCOATS

A classic gentleman's overcoat should be suitable to wear with a formal suit, relaxing over a sweater and jeans, and with a tuxedo for a special event. Few men can afford either the choice or the space for several coats. If you decide that you do want several coats, consider the primary functions of each design before purchasing.

Tip *Exaggerated fashion style coats, even at sale prices, are never a good investment since they are by definition styles of the season.*

CHESTERFIELD This is the classic coat for businesswear. It is a straight-cut and single-breasted coat, with a short vent at the back, knee length, and with a fly front (that is, the buttons concealed by a fold of fabric over the buttoning). The special feature is the chesterfield collar, the cuffs and, in some styles, the pocket flaps. These are made in velvet, either exactly matching the color of the body of the coat, or in a tonal shade such as dark brown with camel, or midnight blue on navy. The fabric of the coat is generally top-quality wool with a plush surface or possibly cashmere and wool or—for true luxury—100 percent cashmere. This coat is especially suited to be worn over a dinner suit or a tuxedo as well as a suit. From time to time fashion has dictated that the chesterfield coat may be double-breasted, especially in the early 60s when it took on a fitted Victorian aspect favored by Teddy Boys, and the 80s when the coat was oversized and boxy to cover the exaggerated shoulder line of that unfortunate sartorial decade.

Tip Try coats on when you are wearing an outfit as close as possible to that which the coat will normally be worn over. That way you may be sure of its practical application.

Left: *A well-cut overcoat should work worn over a suit. This example is versatile and classic enough to wear over a tuxedo, or even a sweater and jeans for city weekends.*

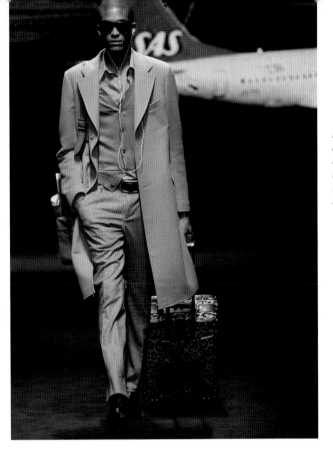

Left: *A classic camel-colored, Crombie-style coat; this will take any businessman anywhere in the world with style and class.*

CROMBIE This is another straight-cut, knee-length coat with a short vent and fly fastening; but the Crombie is always single-breasted and never decorated. This coat tends to be made in heavier-weight wool than the chesterfield. The basic simple streamlined shape can be transformed by designers using a dazzling range of colors and fabrics.

TRENCH The classic raincoat style, especially from Burberry or Aquascutum in London, this typically British coat can be either in wool as an overcoat or in weatherproofed fabric as a raincoat. The style is essentially a belted coat usually with yoke detailing across the shoulders and some fullness of cut. The coat may be knee length or longer depending on the fashion and design.

RAGLAN A roomy easy coat especially suited to go over country clothes with its raglan-cut sleeves. This coat is often made in a textured or tweedy fabric that emphasizes the rustic aspect of the design.

COVERT COAT This coat comes in fine country fabrics in colors ranging from pale beige to leafy greens. It is characterized by three rows of stitching at the cuff and the narrowness of the cut which almost converts it into a jacket on some wearers. There is a velvet collar as on the chesterfield, but this is often colored to tone with the speckled fabric of the coat. Surprisingly for a coat in country shades and a slightly tweedy fabric, this coat is also a classic business coat.

CARRYING CASES

The basic carrying case should be in a dark color, such as black or brown and, if possible in sturdy leather. The case should be the best quality you can afford since, if it is to withstand regular use, it should be well and sturdily constructed from the finest materials. Keep the case polished with colorless leather polish, store it in its original dust bag when not in use, and tidy the contents at regular intervals. All these measures will make sure that the investment you have made in the case has not been wasted. Arriving for an appointment with a greasy backpack or a battered, half-closed bag disgorging its contents will not create a favorable impression.

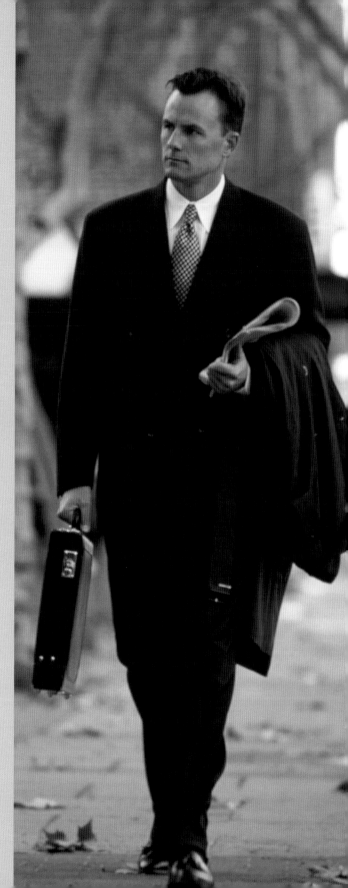

Right: *Finishing touches can make or break an outfit. The bag you carry can say as much about you as your suit. Top to toe means every element of your outfit, as here, should be in harmony.*

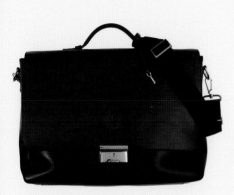

Above: An optional shoulder strap gives this classic briefcase a twist, making it ideal for travel when you have other luggage or bags to carry.

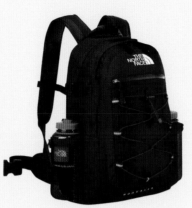

Above: Strictly practical, sporty and relaxed, the backpack should be your second-choice bag for town and business.

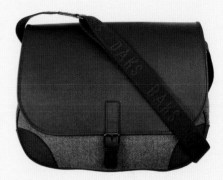

Above: The messenger bag for town must be stylish, classic, and of top quality; it can then become an acceptable variation for business.

Whatever route you take to your place of work, and whatever business papers and equipment you carry around, you need a suitable case to carry them. It should reflect your attitude to your professional conduct and the care you take over detail.

BRIEFCASES Styles may be slim, expandable, or oversize, depending on your needs. There will be a solid handle and, on some cases, a shoulder strap. The number of outside pockets and inside divisions may vary. It should always be able to hold everything you need in general day-to-day business and you should bear this in mind when purchasing a briefcase. You will always create an un-businesslike impression if you are unable to close your bag because of files and papers stuffed in, regardless of the actual capacity of the case.

DOCUMENT CASES These are flat, portfolio-style cases without handles or straps. This style is excellent for papers but unsuited to being crammed with objects. Document cases come in a variety of fabrics, from leather and skins to canvas, and the fastening is either a zipper or fold-over. There are now notepad-style cases with the notepad, pen, and other equipment such as calculators fitted inside them. Approach these with caution: they can look cheap and lazy, a little like a pre-packaged office kit.

Tip A selection of work bags of varying sizes and types not only prolongs the life of each bag but also gives you options.

BACKPACKS For many men, these are the ideal work bag with their many compartments, pockets, and easy straps

to throw over the shoulder, as well as their casual, workmanlike appearance. However, they are not suitable if you wish to appear professional, giving as they do the impression of sporty untidiness. Preferably, they should be reserved for weekends.

MESSENGER BAGS In recent years the idea of the large messenger bag slung diagonally across the body or over the shoulder has introduced a town bag variation, particularly among younger city workers. In leather, nylon and leather, or canvas and leather, these bags combine ease with a more formal style when made of top-quality materials. If you decide to purchase one, consider two things: the bag should be of top quality to avoid looking too casual and sporty, and it should always be worn with a buttoned jacket, to avoid untidiness.

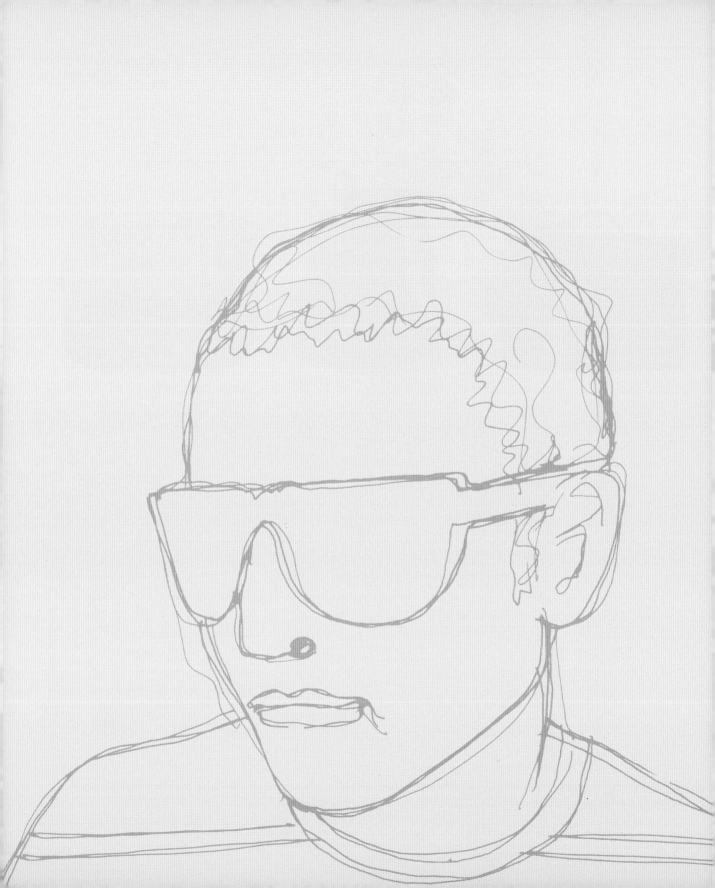

"A woman may sometimes be forgiven for being too stylishly dressed, but a man who looks like a fashion plate is unbearable. Elegant, yes. Foppish, no!"

GENEVIEVE ANTOINE DARIAUX,
AUTHOR AND FASHION DIRECTOR

CITY WEEKEND

The weekend wardrobe for a city resident must be different in content from that of a true country dweller, or even that of the urban resident who has a weekend retreat a short distance from town. Lunch with friends, a visit to a gallery, shopping with your partner, even dinner at a restaurant, are all likely events for the city casual wardrobe, and quite different in dress code from visiting a country fair, strolling on the riverside, or having drinks with friends in a rustic inn.

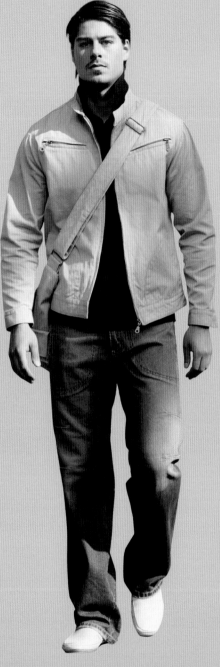

The color choices and fabrics may, at times, overlap with country casual, but the aim of the gentleman who weekends in town is to reflect style and fashion rather than dress for the function of the occasion. Of course, like all contemporary style, the rules are less rigid than ever before and fashion moves on; even the seemingly timeless and classic can create traps for the unwary. Applying the word "safe" to an item or outfit may ultimately turn out to be a synonym for dated. As always, the aim of the gentleman is to be appropriate and stylish in his dress. Urban casual attire is a question of combinations and the key to successful casual dressing in town is to consider the occasion. Ball games in the park with children would obviously be much more casual than shopping in town followed by lunch.

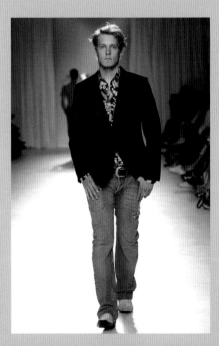

Above: *In this example, formal (the smart jacket) combines with workwear (the straight-leg jean), and city casual (the floral shirt).*

Above: *A simple jacket with clean lines is worn with faded jeans and accessorized with a messanger bag to create the perfect outfit for downtown relaxation.*

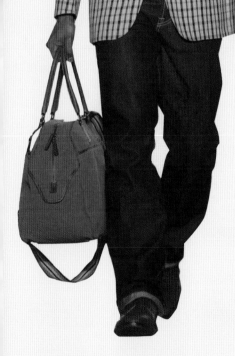

COORDINATED COLOR Jacket, trousers, shirt, and sweater are the four key items, so by selecting a color palette you can give them a well-coordinated look without too much effort. Simply work out the key color for your casual wardrobe, perhaps relating it to your formal clothing; for example, if navy suits are your staple at work, then some navy knitwear, dark indigo jeans, a dash of purple-shaded blues and accents of ice blue or even bright blue, and the casual wardrobe can take a smart jacket into the mix. As another example, if your suits tend to dark gray, this gives you the opportunity to go for "dirty" denim, soft gray knitwear, and accents of paler shades such as lavender and soft sage green.

JACKETS In recent years we have seen a return to formality for men, especially in the city. The concept of the classic single-breasted jacket worn with jeans, or jeans-cut trousers, reflects a new style in urban dressing. The casual jacket may also come in black or dark brown leather; black, navy, or rich dark-colored corduroy; or as a suit jacket teamed with casual pieces. You may select a jacket as classic as you like, with simple clean styling or a more designer version with quirky details, depending on your personal style. These will work with a diverse range of casual items in combinations that cover a variety of excursions, events, and locations.

Above: As shown here, a dash of color, a smart tailored jacket, and a high-quality weekend bag are a winning combination for casual, but smart, style.

CASUAL TOWN JACKETS Jackets, windbreakers, and parkas are among the styles for evenings and weekends. The popularity and fashion of these styles will vary, but generally speaking they are timeless styles which, although varied in silhouette, are still reliable as key pieces for the casual wardrobe.

Tip If a casual parka or windbreaker is to be worn over a tailored jacket, make certain the outer layer is long enough to cover the jacket underneath.

Below: Classic "preppy" style is a timeless variation of menswear pieces that create a sporty and relaxed image. The layers are comprise quality classic items mixed to suit the season and the occasion.

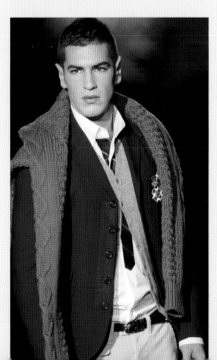

SWEATER AND JEANS

Smart casual is a style oxymoron. If you are looking smart, how can you be casual? The answer is often simple: sweater and jeans teamed with stylish accessories. However, the sweater should be top quality and the jeans should be carefully selected.

CITY CASUAL KNITWEAR For the city, classic simple sweaters in fine wool or cashmere always work and can be varied by the neck shape. A neat crew or V-neck worn under a jacket gives an easy but stylish look

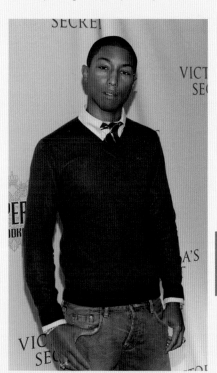

for weekend dressing in town. Remember that fashion will dictate whether turtleneck sweaters may be worn under formal jackets for a more casual look. Strong colors or patterns may be introduced as a statement with urban knitwear, but remember that your friends will notice every time you wear the statement sweater. In winter it can be stylish to wear a chunky knit sweater with more formal clothing to create a town-and-country look. This can be accessorized with a hat, scarf, or gloves for urban winter sports, either participating or simply watching. Never wear knitted hat, scarf, gloves, and sweater: this is knitwear overkill! Break the look up with leather gloves, a fabric scarf, or woven cap.

Tip *When purchasing a sweater, make sure that the shape is flattering and stylish. Slim fit or baggy are the two most stylish variations.*

Left: This slim sweater worn with a shirt and tie is a classic with a twist. **Right:** Stylish but not scruffy, a slouchy soft-shape sweater with easy-fit jeans. **Far right:** Check out the denim of the moment, patchworked (as here) or perhaps a new shade.

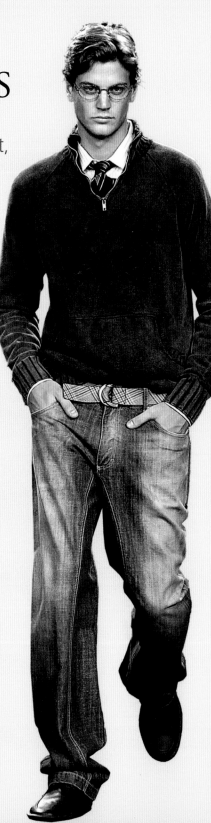

CITY CASUAL JEANS City casual jeans are another contradiction in terms, yet an important item for the casual wardrobe in town. By definition a man's workwear or purely practical garment, jeans are now a designer statement and a recognized part of fashion.

Urban jeans must follow fashion and be updated at regular intervals. You should be aware of changes in shape, color, and detail to ensure that if jeans are to be worn you have selected them from your wardrobe for a purpose and not just pulled a pair on through laziness.

Jeans with the designer label reflect the industry's awareness of the consumer's need to combine garment practicality with a more considered style and image for the city. In the country or suburbs, jeans can be purely practical and worn for the purpose for which they were intended; however, this is patently not true of jeans worn with a smart shirt and jacket to a gallery opening. Baggy and low-rise, boot-cut or ripped and patched, whatever the styles of the moment, you should check them out and watch and discuss. Of all the items guaranteed to make you look outdated, unstylish, and inappropriate, jeans in the city are probably the key danger item.

Tip *Check out the jeans worn by hot new bands; this will tell you what key shapes and shades of denim are being worn.*

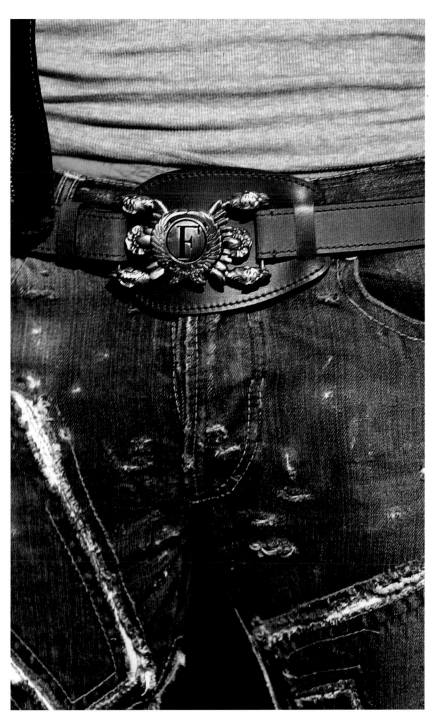

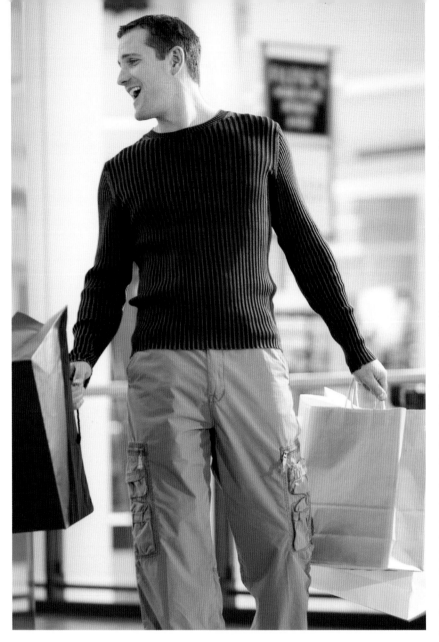

KHAKIS AND SHIRTS

Military styling continues to influence men's fashion. The influence of the practicality and function of the design with the sharp lines and masculine mood combines a confident air with contemporary style.

KHAKIS Tradition plays a large part in menswear style and the development of new rules, developed over the last century, are still based on classic items or concepts used in new ways. Appropriating garments intended for one specific purpose and occasion to another, often diametrically opposed, area of image is no longer a surprise. Military and safari styles developed for active service and practicality were once far removed from fashion and leisure.

In a range of styles, from simple slim jeans to multi-pocketed designs, the khaki pant is a staple of the casual wardrobe. Not even the chino can match its versatility. Khaki as a concept adapts into jackets and vests as well as shirts, largely because it comes in a range of fabric weights and in tones from neutral beige, dark palm green, to prints including camouflage. Finally, there are variations to suit the seasons from a dark khaki wool trench to a soft sand linen shirt. The chino compares with khaki for classic casual pants and for boardwalk shorts, again often with a safari/military style in the detailing and pockets, but cannot compete with the variety and potential of khaki.

Casual in town takes khaki and teams it with a variety of clean-cut pieces to present a modern mix. The items may be a simple pair of easy-cut khaki pants or a designer-led look with an unstructured trench jacket, a multi-pocketed vest, or a simple slim-cut shirt. Common to all these items is practicality and versatility.

CITY CASUAL SHIRTS The important consideration here is not only the color, fabric, and shape, but how the garment is worn. Even some formal shirts can be transformed if worn without a tie, over a T-shirt, or teamed with casual pieces. In style, a city casual shirt should have a less-structured collar, button cuffs, and a more-relaxed fabric. Solid color shirts can cover a spectrum of color, depending on your personal style preferences and the fabric. Pattern with a spot, geometric, stripe, or check is also an option, but always avoid basic lumberjack checks and traditional Hawaiian patterns in town. Shirts with embroidered panels, motifs, or pleats have gained in popularity; they are usually best in self color rather than contrast. The Western shirt or the guyabera (Mexican ruffle) is too much of a specific statement of time and place and should be avoided. Collarless shirts with a slightly Edwardian style may come and go in fashion terms, but are a great classic style for some men.

Chambray is an option, but even this great classic swings in and out of style and the shape and detailing transform over the seasons, so be careful of hanging on to this old faithful casual-shirt fabric.

Short sleeves are problematic; they can be dated in appearance depending on their width and the body shape of the shirt, and, for the purposes of casual wear, which is multifunctional in terms of social events, they can look too dressed down for town. It is far easier to roll sleeves up or down for either climatic or sartorial purposes.

Above all, the city casual shirt is the bridge between the formal shirt you wear for business and your leisure shirt for country, sports, or vacation.

Tip Solid dark colors for casual shirts, although classic, can drain your skin tone and make you look tired. Try dark prints, mid-tones, and sharper colors instead.

CITY CASUAL SHOES
Loafers, brogues, and boots provide a great choice of footwear for casual in town. Sneakers are perfectly fine, but can look too casual for many occasions in town. Jeans teamed with a boot or a heavier lace-up shoe, a formal jacket, and a stylish shirt combine formal and casual with panache.

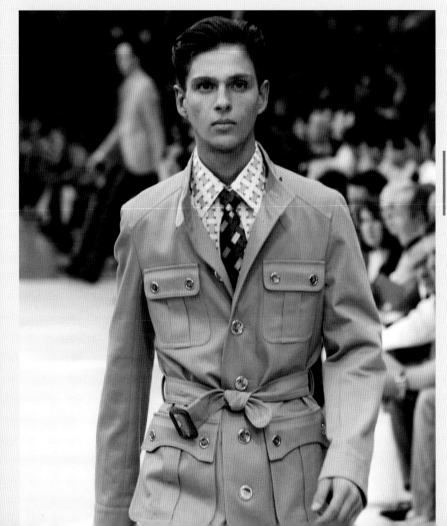

Left: A safari look combines with trench styling for this jacket, here worn with a shirt and tie for smarter weekend occasions. Far left: Classic khaki pants in a combat style work well with neat items like this sweater.

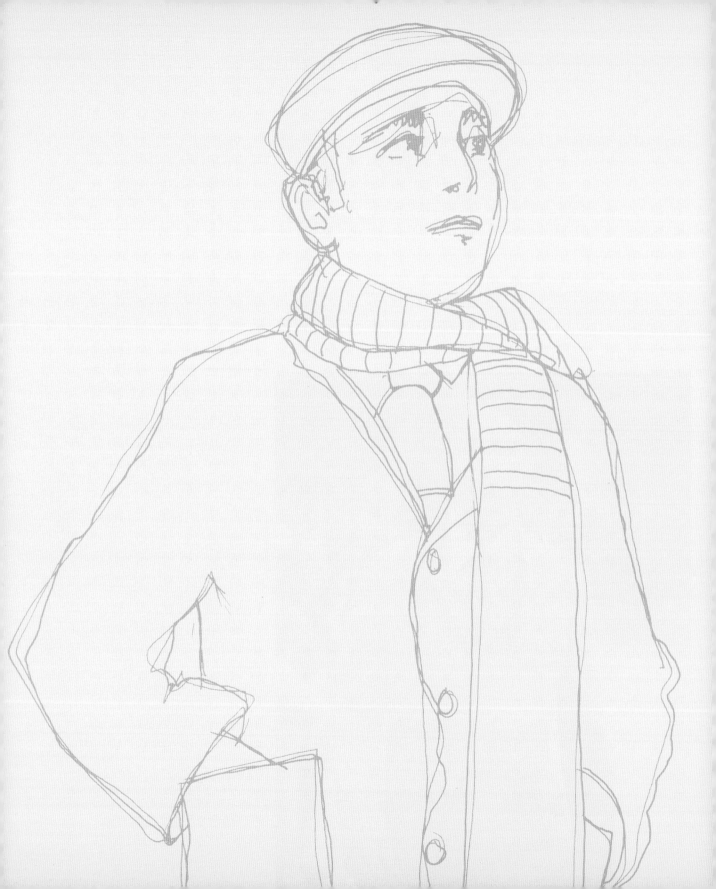

"A ranch hand wears dungarees because they're practical for roping cattle, not because of the way they look; an English country gentleman wears flannels and tweeds because they are suited to his climate; a fisherman, a golfer, or a huntsman wears the gear appropriate to his sport."

HOLLY BRUBACH, FASHION WRITER AND FORMER STYLE EDITOR OF THE NEW YORK TIMES

COUNTRY WEAR

COUNTRY ATTIRE

Harmony of color and texture is key to country attire. If black is urban, it follows that the earth colors are the most rustic. Jackets, collared shirts, and knitwear are fairly standard country wear.

FABRIC When selecting a jacket suitable for the country, we must first look at suitable fabrics. Soft fabrics like moleskin and corduroy (*see Trousers for the Country, page 102*) are suitable, but are for between-season wear and generally more suited for country towns than for outdoor pursuits. Tweed is the hardiest, toughest, and most classic fabric for a country jacket. The weight of tweed has become lighter over the last half-century, but the dense weave and the natural colors of the wool make it the ideal fabric for a classic jacket. Patterns in tweed can vary enormously, from a traditional check in rich autumnal tones to a soft, shaded tweed with an almost feather-like weave, which acts as camouflage amid greenery and shrubs. Specialty shops will stock a wide range of tweed jackets and advise on the suitability for either spectator or sportswear.

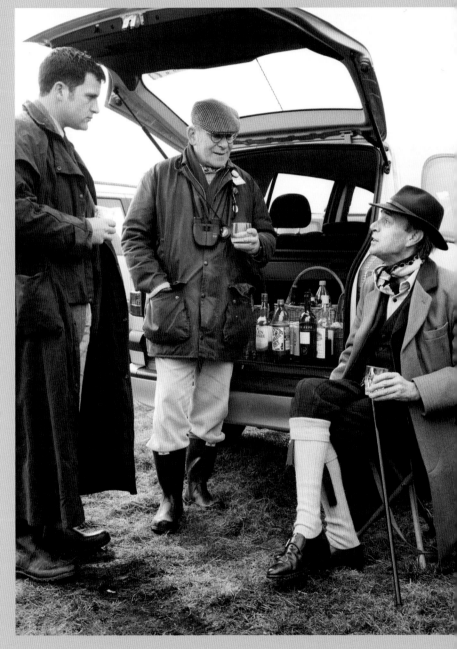

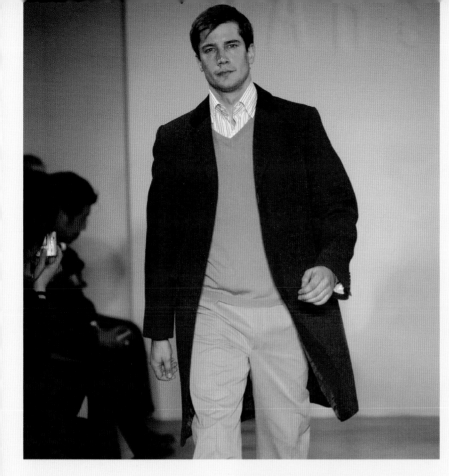

Left: *This Crombie coat takes on a country air by being re-colored. Teamed with easy pieces in the autumnal palette and with soft fabrics, it makes a truly smart country statement.*

BLAZER A casual double-breasted flannel jacket with patch pockets developed in the 1890s and worn for boating, cricketing, and seaside pursuits. Versions may be plain or striped and often with a club or team crest on the breast pocket and brass buttons, which may also feature a team motif.

WEATHERPROOF JACKETS & COATS
Depending on the kind of country weekend you or your host have planned, a weatherproof garment can be a lifesaver. Rainproof, windproof, and well-lined jackets and coats will protect you against the elements. Lightweight weatherproofed jackets using advanced fabrics are a good investment and if they can be carried in a bag until required, so much the better.

STYLE Jackets for the country will be single-breasted with patch-style pockets or a mix with pockets featuring button-over flaps, bellows (a pocket with extra fabric between the pocket and the body of the garment), or even zippers. All pockets are for function and practicality, rather than decoration or fashion whim. Country jackets are often cut surprisingly narrow, but have extra fabric around the armhole to allow for freedom of movement. Unnecessary bulk in country clothes is not part of the style, since they are traditionally designed for activity.

Tip Country pursuits often involve many hours away from home; make sure you have allowed for weather changes during the time you are out.

LEATHER & SUEDE The practicality and toughness of leather and suede lend themselves to country clothing and are often used for trimmings and details, from knotted leather buttons on a jacket to suede panels on jodhpurs. Sheepskin jackets and coats in a wide range of lengths are also classic, but they should always be straightforward in style: nothing over-designed works in the country. Leather jackets, either in classic blouson style or in a simple basic jacket shape, are appropriate, but ensure that they are not black—not a color for a gentleman's country wardrobe.

Tip Tweed jackets are classic and useful to have in your wardrobe. If you see an excellent example on sale, it is well worth purchasing.

TOP COATS The two most suitable styles of coat for the country are the raglan coat and the classic trench. Color must be sympathetic to the country surroundings and the garments should be classic. If your weekend is dressier, then the covert coat will be appropriate for mixing in with classic country weekend items. (*See Business Coats, page 87.*)

TROUSERS FOR THE COUNTRY

It is a perceived tradition among many city dwellers that any old clothes will do for the country. Not only is this a misapprehension, it can lead to serious misdressing. Country trousers may not have the crisp finish of the city suit trouser, but the variety of fabrics and styles offers very stylish options, even staying close to classic country traditions. Rich textures and colors open up new clothing opportunities as well as giving those trousers endlessly worn in the city a rest.

CORDUROY Literally "the king's cord," corduroy is a fabric favored for both town and country and is historically linked to the country for both jackets and trousers. The corduroy suit has a softly tailored edge, which seems entirely appropriate for formal rustic occasions, while corduroy jackets or trousers teamed with tweeds and knitwear bring to mind images of oak-beamed taverns and discussions of livestock. Corduroy is described by the number per inch of its "wales," the ribs of pile woven onto the plain background. Wales vary from finest needlecord, suitable even for shirts, to elephant cord, which is in truth more suitable for upholstery. Although made of cotton, corduroy is essentially a winter fabric since the density of the construction makes it warm.

There are two color groups appropriate to corduroy: the rich club shades of claret, bottle green, and navy blue, and the autumnal tones of gold, pumpkin, heather, and peat.

Tip Waterproof trousers are very much part of country activities, but they are not versatile and should only be worn out of doors, whereas all other country trousers may be worn on a variety of occasions and dressed up with a jacket or down with a sweater.

Left: Practical, comfortable, and stylish; this outfit is based around a sweater, jacket, and trousers, yet it has real impact due to the color and fabric combinations which reflect the influence of the country in tone and texture.

COUNTRY TROUSERS Alongside corduroy are several other styles and fabrics suitable for a variety of country occasions and pursuits. Interestingly, they are predominantly cotton fabrics with a weave or surface adding warmth.

Cavalry twill and whipcord fabrics are characterized by a distinctive diagonal rib on the surface of the fabric, making them both hard-wearing and practical. Both fabrics tend to come in cream, buff, and other neutral shades.

Moleskin, as its name implies, has a soft velvety surface like the fur of a mole. This fabric lends itself to muted colors that blend in with the countryside.

Heavy military-style khakis (*see Khakis and Shirts, page 97*) may also be worn in the country, especially in weatherproofed or woolen fabrics.

Tweeds for trousers are either specific in their sporting usage (hiking or shooting) or worn as part of a suit. Tweed trousers cropped to just below the knee and sometimes fastened with a buckle are called plus fours, and can be wonderful on the correct occasion. Tweed is generally preferred for jackets and coats since it is rough, thus requiring lining, yet soft, which means it loses its shape with wearing very quickly.

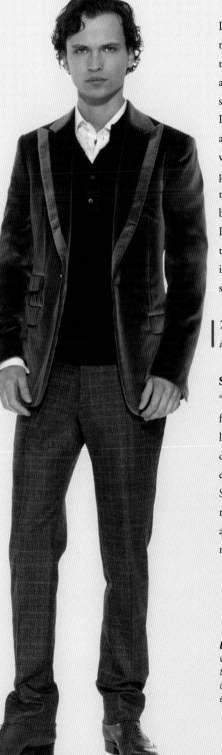

Like all sports, country sports from golfing to shooting and fishing require specific trouser styles. Many country sport trousers are designed to be worn with longer, thicker socks and either boots or heavy shoes. If invited to participate in any specialized activity, be sure to ascertain what your host will be wearing and whether he will be providing suitable clothing for you and the other guests or whether you need to borrow or rent an outfit for the event. If you have no intention of either taking up the particular pursuit, or ever participating in it again, there is no need to purchase specialized clothing.

Tip For horseback riding, the correct attire is always jodhpurs and boots.

SUMMER COUNTRY TROUSERS
"Easy fit" characterizes summer trousers for the country, lending itself in style to linen and softer fabrics. Pleated front or drawstring waist and clean uncluttered details work well for this style of trouser. Summer trousers for the country may be rolled up for waterside activities such as rowing, thus giving a relaxed edge to more formal looks.

Left: *The color creates a country house dandy with this velvet jacket. Bordering on the style of creative dressing, this is an Edwardian, possibly even Victorian, image updated for a traditional country weekend candlelit evening or dinner.*

KNITWEAR

There are several basic things to know about knitwear before you purchase a garment. Much of the terminology for knitwear comes from the British Isles, where knitwear has a long heritage and tradition. Knitwear is constructed of yarn, and what the yarn is made of will affect the feel of the garment. The main yarn types are Shetland (a hairy, rustic yarn), lambs' wool (softer and finer), merino (the softest and finest wool from sheep), and finally, cashmere (which comes from goats and is generally the finest and the softest yarn to knit with).

The weight of the yarn depends upon the number of threads that are twisted together to make the yarn, starting with fine two-ply and increasing to bulkier and fatter yarns. Patterns come in two major styles, either integral to the knit (such as a classic Fair Isle, jacquard, or intarsia) or as raised surface texture (found in cables, ribs, or Arran knits).

Tip *Be sure to check the latest fashion for knitwear, because nothing ages you like your father's old Christmas cardigan!*

When it comes to the shape and type of garment in style, there are many variations combining all the elements from yarn to stitch. Bear in mind the overall style of the garment itself: is it a sweater, polo shirt, cardigan, or pullover? Is it "fully fashioned," meaning the garment is shaped as it is made, or is it cut out and sewn together? The most important consideration is the shape of the sweater—compare it with contemporary fashion. Is it slim cut, boxy, or pulled in by a heavily ribbed knitted band finishing off the cuffs and hem? These design elements change over the seasons. At present, a sweater should be slim but straight with no emphasis on the rib; in fact, many modern sweaters are hemmed at the bottom with no rib.

Tip *Not all yarn is suitable for gentlemen: there is an edited selection suitable for menswear garments.*

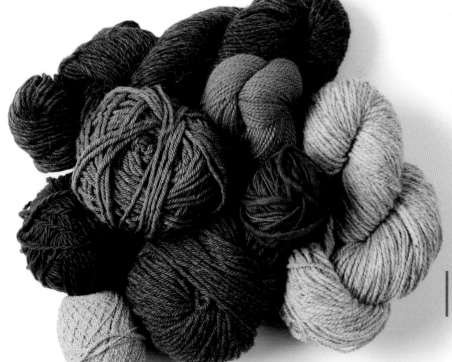

Since knitwear tends to cling, the sweater's shape needs careful thought. For example, a deep V-neck flatters a short or wide neck, while sloping shoulders can be offset by a fully fashioned sleeve. It is therefore advisable to try all knitwear on before purchasing as well as taking into account what the sweater may be worn with—either under (perhaps a T-shirt), or over (maybe a slim jacket).

Now put all the elements together, add pattern, and you will see how complex selecting a suitable sweater can become. Don't panic, though. There are simple steps to help you choose the appropriate knitwear.

Classic fine quality sweaters will fit under tailored jackets and mix with a variety of looks. Chunky knit and rustic sweaters work mainly in the country, but can also look stylish in the city with jeans, a tailored jacket, and classic brogues. Knit polo shirts with long sleeves can make a formal suit look relaxed, as can cardigans. Cardigans go in and out of style and, like other types of knitwear, can be aging and convey a comfortable, settled image. The key to a successful knitwear purchase is to spend time with style magazines and check the leading fashion retailers for their views on knitwear at that particular moment.

Above right: This cool white sweater can be worn skiing or sailing, it has such quality and style.
Right: The soft camouflage sweater, shown here in natural tones, is versatile for country wear, and will work with corduroy, denim, or military-style pant.

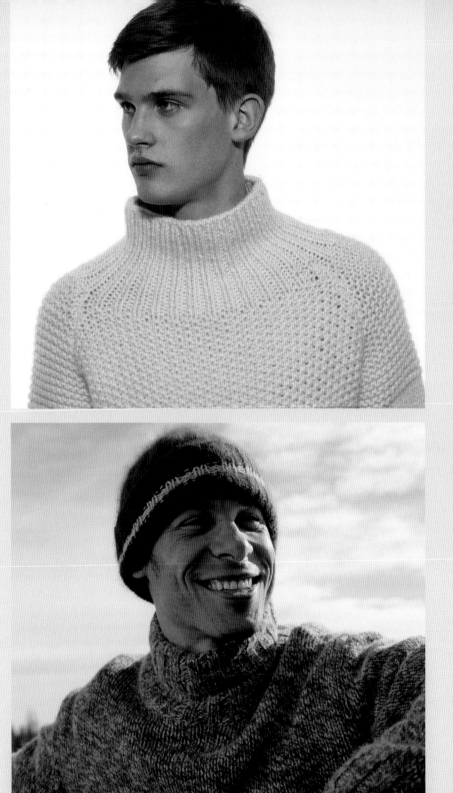

KNITWEAR

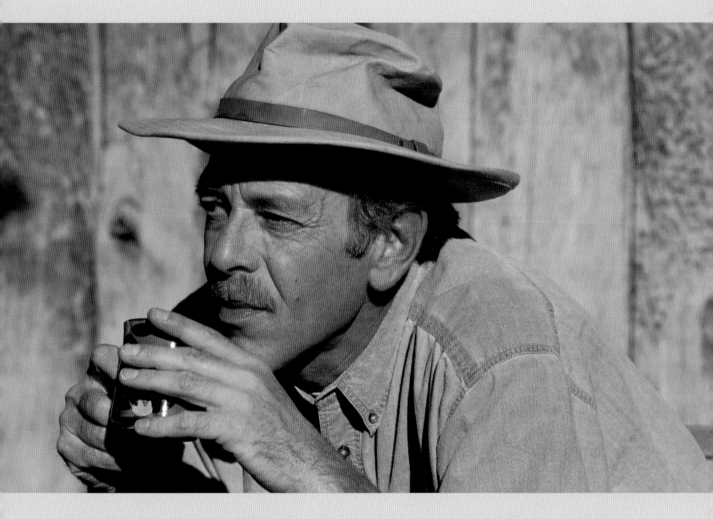

SHIRTS FOR THE COUNTRY

COUNTRY WEAR

The country, either in summer or winter, can be surprisingly formal. Tradition has made a firm impression on country clothing, so do not run away with the idea that a denim shirt and a T-shirt or two will do. The country shirt is less structured in all senses than a formal town shirt, but it should, as always, be of top quality, stylish but understated, as befits a gentleman.

Just because you are no longer in the city does not mean you can go wild with decorative patterns and bold color; in fact, shirt patterns are limited in the country. Classic country shirts often come in checks such as Tattersall, reflecting the importance of the equestrian world in country life, or windowpane. Avoid the lumberjack-style plaid shirt over a T-shirt look; while it is classic, it is not appropriate for a weekend of hiking and sightseeing. Likewise, Western shirts with multicolored embroidery will only work if you are a cowboy.

COLLARLESS SHIRTS The addition of the collarless shirt, originally a vintage item, to the country wardrobe started in the 70s, when hippy and caftan styles became popular. Although the collarless shirt can be a great item for informal weekends or on vacation, when it can be teamed with a drawstring trouser to create an almost unstructured suit look, the collarless style does not suit all body types. The narrow-band collar combined with the easy-fit shape, usually made of washed cotton and often styled with a tuxedo front of soft pleats, can be unflattering to a larger man. The best advice is to try on several styles before purchasing, but it is also possible that, although classic, this particular item is not for you.

COUNTRY SHIRTS For summer formal country events, shirts in candy stripes, which one could never wear in town, can work with a plain dark blazer. This is also the time and place for floral shirts to

become a modern classic. They are best in a slim shape and when neatly printed all over with medium-sized flowers in a matching range of colors; for example, all pinks or all yellows rather than rainbow. However, soft plain fabrics characterize the country shirt, often with brushed surfaces or textural weaves. The country shirt should always be in complementary tones to your tweeds and corduroys. The country shirt will have a softer collar and usually button cuffs, and the shape will be easy in fit to allow for an active, outdoor life. In summer, linen shirts in white, ivory or extremely pale colors, cut in a classic formal style, can be worn.

COUNTRY TIES The motifs and fabrics for ties worn in the country can be quite different from even an urban casual tie. Woven ties in heavy fabrics, even wool, often with plaid or tartan as the motif, are classic with country shirts, as are silk ties with equestrian or other sporting insignia. Conversational prints such as small paisleys or stylized flowers are also popular for country ties. Colors tend to reflect the rustic or club palette with green predominating in a range of vegetation-based shades. Tie clips and pins also appear more often in the country setting to restrain the tie during physical activities.

Tip Some country clubs and restaurants are surprisingly formal, so always take ties to the country and check if you are unsure of the form.

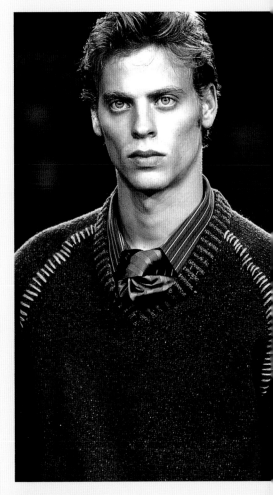

Above: *Even worn with a tie this shirt is country in style and coloring, especially when worn under a rustic sweater.*
Far left: *Washed and weathered shirts take color to the country, but in strictly practical fabrics and styles.*

COUNTRY WORKWEAR

While it may seem that all you need for the country is jeans and a sweater, jeans are not always the best option. Denim is a tough workwear fabric, but there are plenty of other options, for both trousers and jackets. When looking at the items and style of the country wardrobe, there are many more suitable options that can give your image a modern yet classic look.

Right: *Jeans are transformed into country essentials when teamed with rustic checks and practical accessories for the great outdoors.*

DENIM If you decide to wear denim in the country, make certain of a number of elements when selecting the items. First, do not choose a fashionable style; go for classic easy fit and practicality. The jeans you wear in the country should not have rips which get caught in every passing branch, have flares which drag in the mud, or be so tight they restrict movement. Classic jeans in traditional workable shapes are what are required. The same applies to a denim jacket: no fancy fashion details or embellishments are required in the country. If you are asked to engage in such activities as shifting hay, digging ground, or simply walking some distance, you do not need to be wearing clothing that prevents this.

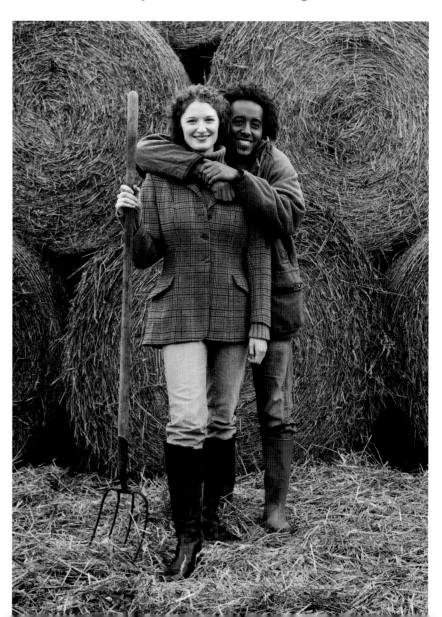

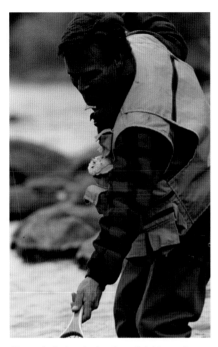

Above: A gilet is a timeless item of clothing, and entirely practical for the country.

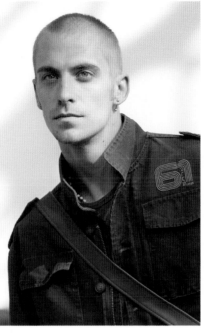

Above: Heavier fabrics in a rich country green are used here for a tough military-styled jacket.

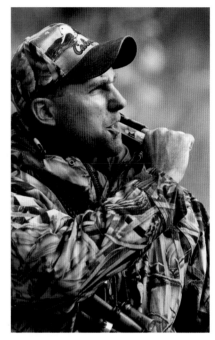

Above: Every activity has its own camouflage wear, whether by the water, as above, or on the land.

GILETS Gilets are useful garments that come in a surprisingly diverse range of styles. A gilet is simply a sleeveless jacket with a zipper, stud, or button fastened front. Since the garment has no sleeves it allows for good arm movement which makes it suitable attire for activities such as fishing. Fabrics cover all types from quilted technical surfaces through to heavy wools and even leather and shearling (sheep's leather that retains the short stubby wool left after shearing intact).

Tip When putting country clothes together, never overstyle, either by matching combinations or with tacky promotional accessories, such as rock band T-shirts.

MILITARY Heavier military-style khakis (*see Khakis and Shirts in page 97*) may also be worn in the country, especially in woolen or wind- or waterproofed fabrics. Brushed wool, or boiled and felted wool (which is as the name suggests: woven wool that is boiled or felted to make it tougher and more compact in texture) can make terrific outerwear. In navy blue or rustic and camouflage greens, military-style garments from a short coat to a gilet are both functional and stylish in the country. Obviously in warmer weather summer khakis and cargo styles also work in the country, but should be styled in a more practical and relaxed way than for town.

CAMOUFLAGE Traditional military camouflage fabric is not always the best option for country weekends, but fabrics with a camouflage aspect to them are different. Muted greens and browns allow the wearer to blend with the countryside, whether just walking and observing or participating in a sporting activity. And, the practical styling of such clothing can be interpreted in many fabrics, so that camouflaged gilets or trousers can be made in brushed cotton or weatherproofed technical fabric.

Tip Never, ever, wear a complete denim outfit unless you really do own a working ranch. Denim overkill is a surefire middle-aged, suburban style hazard.

COUNTRY FOOTWEAR

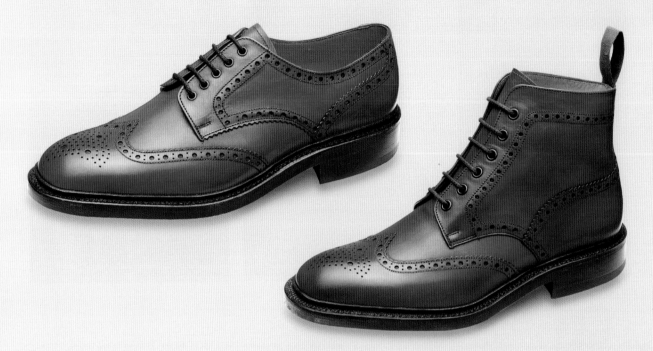

Country activities offer many challenges for footwear, especially if you are usually an urban dweller. Appearing in a pair of brand-new Timberland boots hardly makes you a countryman. Specialized country activities require specialized footwear and it is always advisable to check with your host what is planned for the weekend and whether you need to provide riding boots, tennis shoes, or climbing boots.

SHOES Stout hiking shoes or brogues will see you through most seasons in the country; they balance heavy country fabrics and provide protection for the foot from uneven ground. These shoes should be brown lace-ups with a good stout sole. If well polished before storing, these classic country shoes should last several years. If they need repairs of any sort, make certain this is done before they are put away.

SUMMER SHOES In the summer, deck shoes are versatile for country wear, but do not allow them to become overtired in appearance unless you are a regular sailor. Canvas shoes or leather and canvas shoes in classic lace-up designs are timeless and practical; if you spend much time in the country during the summer it is worth investing in a selection of these more formal summer styles.

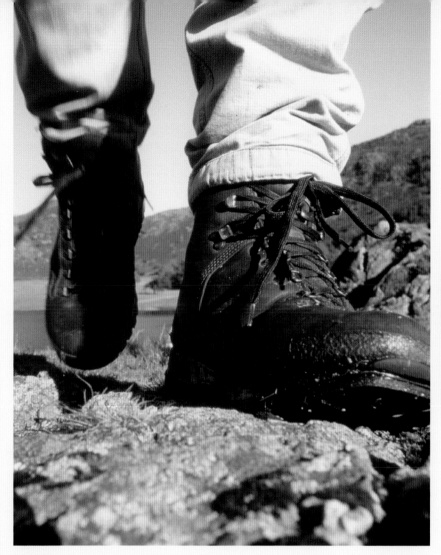

Left: Functional practicality is the key to appropriate country footwear, whether cross-country or mountain hiking. Classic boots and shoes which have built-in protection in their construction and fabrics are always winners for country wear.

Below: Unlike those worn for business, country socks are often colored or patterned.

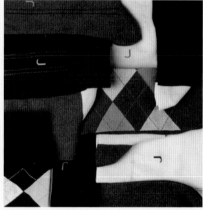

BOOTS Boots come in a wide range of designs and shapes. You are looking for a classic that will work with outdoor clothing for hiking as well as indoor attire, perhaps for lunch or sightseeing. Buy boots of the best quality you can afford, since they are not a fashion item and will also improve with age and wear—this is considered investment dressing. Once purchased, the boots will remain in your closet and, if well cared for, will last many years. Boots come with either eyeholes to lace up or hooks to lace around; either is acceptable and in fact some boots combine both.

A stout boot or shoe, even for an activity seemingly as prosaic as hiking, can be a trap for the unwary. Striding through the countryside in medium-weight town brogues is no substitute for wearing stout walking boots with sturdy soles and proper quality padding in the right places.

Tip If you do not live in the country, the footwear you take on your country visit should have been worn around town to give it a patina and to allow your feet to become accustomed to heavier footwear than you usually put one.

SOCKS Even in warmer weather, stout socks are usually part of country weekend apparel. Make certain you have the correct socks to wear with boots or stout shoes. These will be thick, ribbed, and longer than town socks. Country socks for more regular wear also include the argyle pattern in both rustic and club colors. Summer socks may also include finer weight socks in argyle but in pastel shades. It is also permissible to go without socks with canvas shoes, deck shoes or lightweight loafers in the summer, provided this suits your style and you have well cared-for feet.

Tip Lightweight loafers are an alternative shoe for the country town if you are wearing dark trousers, but under no circumstances wear a heavy town shoe with summer clothing.

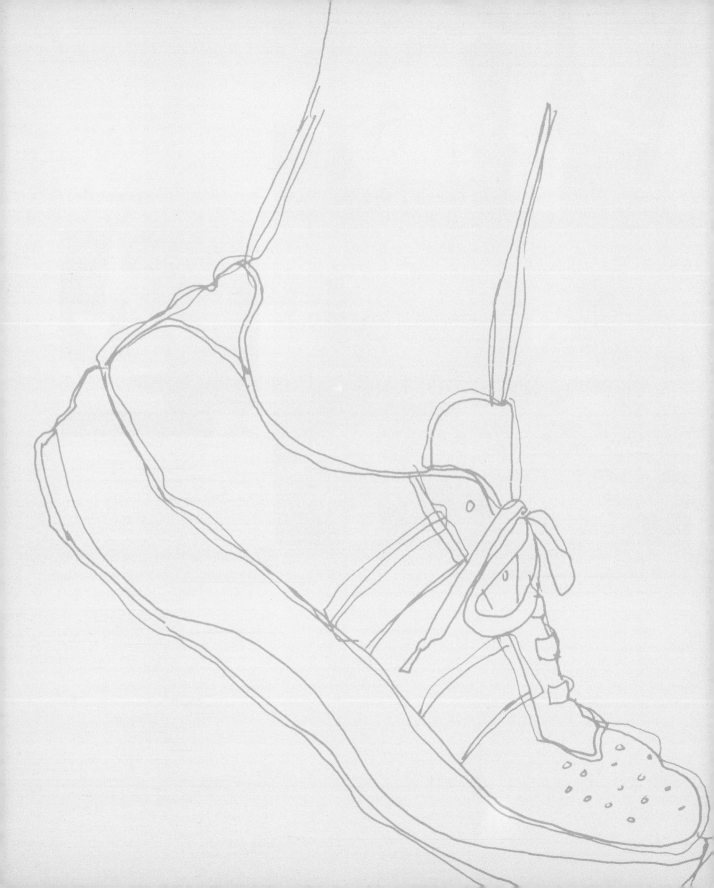

"In the twentieth century sports have been the major influence on fashion. They have liberated fashion by gradually accustoming the eye to new ideas and familiarizing the body to new designs."

FRANCE-MICHELE ADLER, SPORTS FASHION WRITER

THE SPORTING LIFE

Gentlemen's pursuit of sports has a history as ancient as many of the sports themselves. Playing a sport, coaching the players, sponsoring the participants and events, or supporting and spectating, the world of sports is, for many men, much more than an interest or a hobby—it is their life's blood.

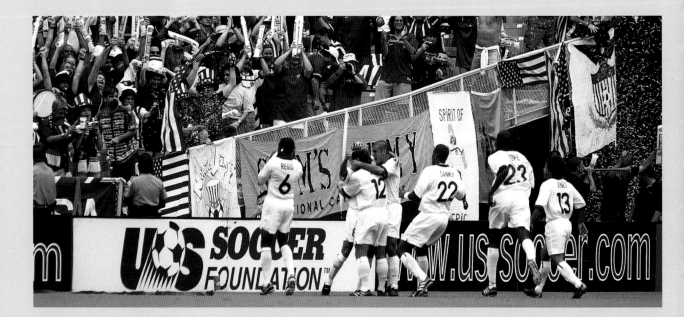

The passions that sports arouse are reflected in the team colors, crest, or uniform; in the rules of when, where, and how to flaunt your team's insignia; even in how to dress to watch the game or match. A gentleman may run the risk of sartorial embarrassment at any time, but the highest risk area is in sports, since the rules are rigid within a specific sport but variable from team to team. Tradition plays an enormous

role within all sports, and the only answer to avoiding local pitfalls is to ask, as this is truly a case of better safe than sorry. Simply because your particular team does it one way, doesn't mean that all teams follow the same procedures, and in fact most teams pride themselves on their idiosyncrasies. So a well-timed and discreetly asked question may save you from more than egg on your face. The advice throughout this section is based on one

simple rule—do your homework. If it is unfamiliar territory, for whatever reason, check, investigate, question, and research before setting off with your inappropriate sweater, tie, or scarf in completely the wrong stripe or colors.

Above: *The influence of style on sportswear is often in the shape. These players are wearing a different version of the teamwear from that of their fathers' and grandfathers' generations.*

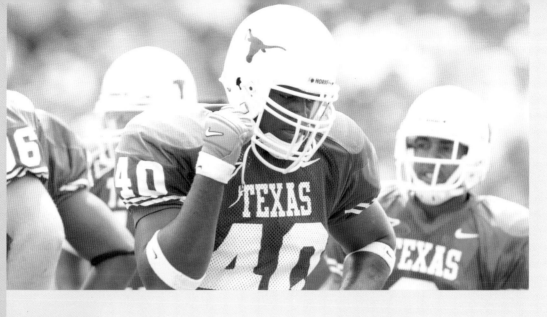

Right: The team spirit underpins all clothing choices in team sports, whether playing or cheering.

Below: Active sport in the city still requires investment in appropriate attire, even if it is simply suitable shorts, T-shirt and shoes, as shown here.

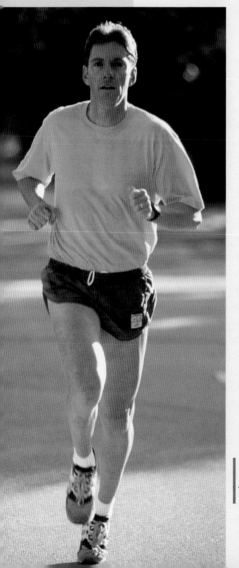

CITY SPORTS

Some typical urban sports include cycling, swimming, tennis, jogging and running, in-line skating and ice skating, boxing, fencing, and bowling. Some of these require minimal equipment and in some cases minimal additional clothing; however, it is important to remember that your effectiveness and success in all sporting activities will be greatly enhanced by suitable attire. It may be suitable footwear, classic jogging pants, or a roomy shirt to allow for freedom of movement. Whatever the specifics, a brief conversation with someone who is an experienced practitioner of the sport will inform you as to the real clothing needs and those that are optional. Many urban sports are pursued indoors, allowing for a change into appropriate attire in changing facilities. Outdoor sports in town are often a weekend pleasure, which means you can leave home ready and dressed for the pavement or park.

Tip Basic active sports pieces tend to be function- rather than fashion-led, so buy good-quality pieces when you find them.

BALL GAMES

Rugby, soccer, football, basketball, hockey, softball, and volleyball are just some of the ball games you are likely to come across, many of these not confined to town but held at a park, stadium, or field that is easily accessible from town. Since ball games are team games, inappropriate colors may constitute a major sartorial faux pas. Watching or participating, it makes no difference in the strength of feeling that team loyalty engenders. Check before joining a game or watching your friends' team play, on any special color to be either celebrated or avoided to show your undying support for the correct side. Within some sports, stripes are part of the team uniform, so again, check before wearing an incorrectly striped tie to the directors' stand at the game.

Tip If you are inexperienced at a sport, it is ill advised to buy top-of-the-line clothing and appear as a first class professional, only to let others down by your obvious lack of prowess.

THE SPORTING LIFE

COUNTRY SPORTS

The perception is that
country sports are
typically English, yet
many country sports
played in America are
of French, Canadian,
or Scottish origin. The
key feature of country
sports is that the clothing
should encompass both
practicality and an
element of camouflage.
Golf, hiking, fishing,
shooting, horseback
riding and show jumping,
polo, camping, climbing,
and mountaineering are
among the most common
country sporting activities.

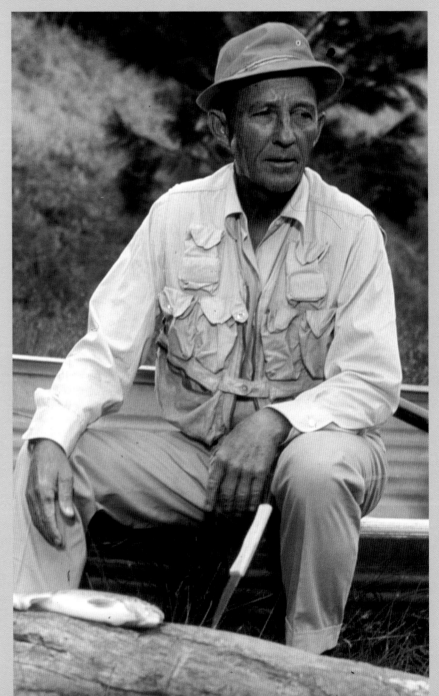

Right: Comfort and
tradition are never out
of style for relaxation,
and practical details add
function not fuss.

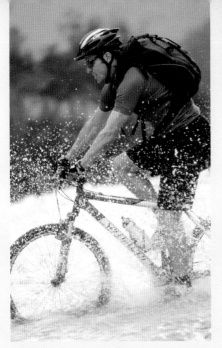

Above: Cycling on all kinds of terrains, with innovative variations on the bicycle itself, is matched with technological bike wear.

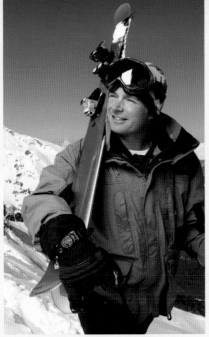

Above: Fashion and style play a very minor part in this strictly practical ski outfit.

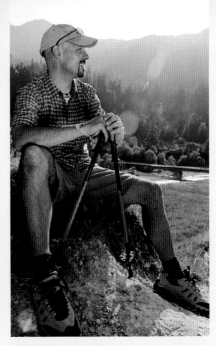

Above: Hiking and climbing call for uncluttered clothing in tough fabrics.

For many country sports, it is of major importance that they rely on tradition; even in this day and age, the rules laid down a hundred or more years ago still apply and it would be foolish to flout convention. Once again, fashion has little to do with sporting attire. Appropriate and practical garments win the day.

COLOR AND FABRIC

Fabric should be strictly practical whatever the sport, but for country sports it should both protect and blend with the great outdoors. For most country sports, the idea is to be invisible to animals, yet be warm and protected. In essence, tweeds and other fabrics are created to merge with the landscape in both texture and coloring. In the case of winter sports, such as skiing, however, you actually wish to be visible to everyone. If some unfortunate accident befalls you, you need to be sure that there is every chance of being seen from a distance.

WINTER SPORTS

Wherever you may be in the world, seasonal sports, and indeed the season of sports, plays an important role in many men's lives. The start of the sporting season, due either to tradition or climatic change, marks a clear change in the lives of many men. There is also an element of travel for specific seasonal sports, especially if snow is involved. For winter sports such as skiing, ice skating, snowboarding, curling, and bobsledding, protective clothing should primarily protect against the cold and also guard against injury. As always with sportswear, the design is determined by the performance of the sport.

Tip Since traditional hunting, shooting, and fishing suppliers will know far more than you on specifics, trust their advice when purchasing clothing from them.

WINTER FOOTWEAR AND ACCESSORIES

It must be noted that, for both winter and country sports, appropriate footwear is essential. Always choose the appropriate footwear for the activity, and do not skimp on good boots. Waterproofing on a boot can save a chill, and proper structure can reduce the possibility of slipping or twisting the foot on uneven terrain.

Since all the climatic elements can be dangerous, it seems invidious to deem winter more treacherous than summer; yet both extremes of cold and heat can, in sporting activities, offer unpleasant surprises to the unwary. It must therefore be noted that if sun protection is essential for summer, it can also be needed for winter. In addition, while you are skiing, your ears can suffer from wind chill and your fingers from frostbite: adequate protection is thus not aesthetic but strictly practical.

SUMMER SPORTS

Swimming, sailing, surfing, water-skiing, rowing, and canoeing are among the water-based sporting activities that are enjoyed during summer. Aside from the specifics, clothing for these sports starts not only with practical application, such as lightweight fabric and construction, but also with consideration of the waterproof quality of these design elements.

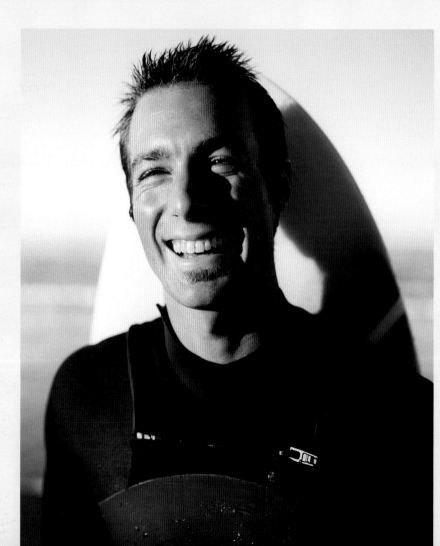

As with most sportswear, the garments are not so much about fashion and seasonal changes as they are about the adaptation of the clothing to the demands of climate, situation, and physical practicalities. Swimsuit, sailing jacket, or wetsuit, each has a function to perform as part of the exercise. Woe betide you if you fail to consider this when purchasing your clothes! Reputable manufacturers—that is, the key names with specialized knowledge—will be stocked by expert outfitters and this is where you should go to shop rather than a fashion boutique.

Tip *Picnic baskets are often a prerequisite for summer sporting events. If you have any doubts as to your expertise, in the long run it is cheaper and less worrisome to purchase one already prepared.*

Left: *A healthy active outdoor sport such as surfing, boarding or jet skiing requires the correct clothes, not just shorts and a T-shirt.*

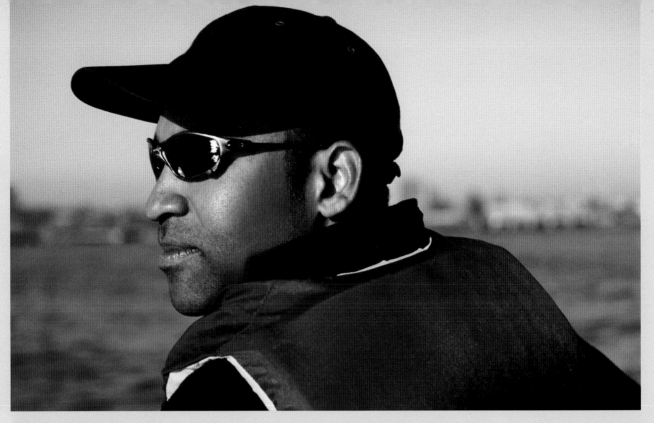

Above: *During the summer hats and shades are not fashion accessories, they are practical protection from the elements. By wearing them you may well save yourself from many uncomfortable hours of eyestrain and sunburn.*

SPECTATOR

Polo, tennis, football, baseball and sailing are among the sports that involve large numbers of spectators at the events. Attending a game, either with a friend or as the guest of a business colleague, can be fraught with sartorial dangers. As mentioned with team sports, colors, stripes, and so on can impart a message of alliance unintended when you dressed for the event. So be wary and check team colors. Also ascertain where you will be watching from, as the dress code for the chairman's stand may differ from standing with the rest of the crowd. Clubhouses often have stringent, not to say draconian, rules as to what members' and guests' attire is considered suitable, so again check on the individual rules; from blazer and tie to anything goes is a fair distance when gauging dress codes. Charity or special events may also shift the sartorial requirements to a higher level of dress for a gentleman. Formal race meetings require much more consideration when dressing than just spending the day at the local races. A certain amount may be gauged from the invitation, but for a gentleman, especially if with a companion, it is always a good idea to check the dress code before such an event.

Tip Umbrellas can double as sun protection on hot days of the year, so don't just view them as bad-weather accessories.

SKIN CARE

Exposure to the relentless effects of the sun, plus water and all its attendant side effects, means that you cannot afford to ignore skin care in either summer sports or water-based activities. When sailing or surfing, the blast from water and sun will dry and redden the skin wherever it is exposed. As an example, if you are balding or have closely cropped hair, the sun will dry your scalp and damage what hair remains. Your nose will become sunburned if not protected and moisturized. Caring for your skin is neither effeminate nor overcautious, but simply a matter of self-preservation and common sense, since a peeling scalp, a bright red nose, or dry, chapped lips are not signs of masculinity but of carelessness and a lack of attention to practicality.

SUMMER SPORTS

SPORTING ACCESSORIES

You should remember that sporting accessories have little to do with fashion but everything to do with practicality. Protection from the elements, hair control, and sweat absorption are more important than style. Sports accessories are often timeless, so invest wisely.

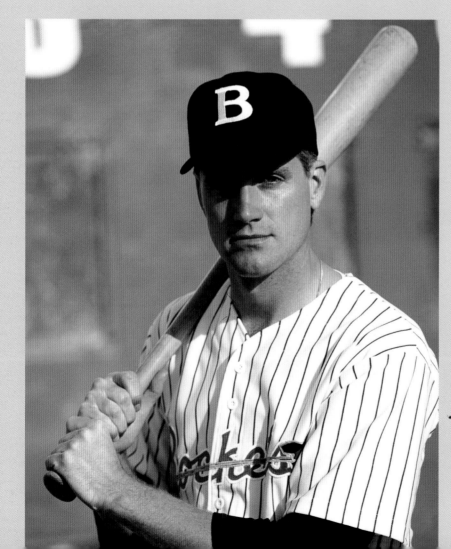

TEAM CLOTHING

Sweatshirts, T-shirts, scarves, and even wristbands may all signal an allegiance to a specific team. These are readily available at the team meet or club and not only indicate your support but also contribute to the team's fundraising. In your enthusiasm to support a team, remember that such items work in other ways as well, such as antagonizing opposing team members or becoming meaningless when worn outside the team area. Finally, there is the aesthetic consideration, which is that, although admirable in their supporting aspect, promotional garments are rarely fashionably of high merit, so be sure you are investing your money wisely before purchasing.

HATS

Whether baseball caps, ski caps, or shooting caps, headwear is widely in evidence in the sporting world, and is usually allied to a specific activity, including team, sponsors, insignia, and slogans. The main reason for wearing hats is as sun protection, and this applies especially to spectators. When you are standing in the sun, a hat becomes essential and not a luxury. A Panama, a soft finely woven straw hat with a dimpled crown and a semi-soft brim, is especially suitable for this purpose in the summer, as is the classic boater, a hard straw hat with a flat circular brim and a ribbon band, often in the colors of a team.

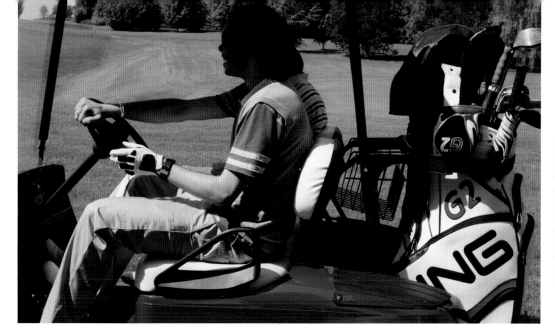

Left: *Gloves can be an important item for certain sporting activities, as here with golf. Protection and practicality are, as ever, the key to their purchase and wearing.*
Far left: *Team garments are rarely stylish, so the discerning gentleman should purchase with caution.*

UMBRELLAS

Umbrellas often come into their own as an accessory, whether you are playing a sport such as golf, or perhaps watching polo or tennis. Large golf umbrellas, some boldly emblazoned with company logos, also double as walking sticks. A small folding umbrella carried with sporting equipment is another accessory with a truly practical application in inclement weather.

SHOES & BOOTS

Finishing touches can make or break your first impression on every occasion. At sporting events, whether cheering your team on or participating yourself, the wrong footwear can completely skew an outfit. Not only the wrong choice of footwear but also brand-new or shiny shoes can mark you as a complete novice who is unaware of the finer points of the game. It is advisable to break in sport boots or shoes well before joining your friends at the event.

SPORT BAGS

Specialized bags for golf clubs or angling equipment give the impression of professionalism and forethought. Apply this concept to any sporting activity, be it in-line skating or regular gym visits, and you have understood that the appropriate tool for the job follows through in all areas of grooming. If you regularly take gym clothes to the office, for example, your sports bag should be discreet and complement your business attire. If you only use a sports bag to go straight to the gym, it can be branded or colored and should be purely practical.

PICNIC BASKETS

Picnic baskets are not an essential part of a gentleman's wardrobe; however, if you are involved in many summer spectator sports, the well-fitted picnic hamper or basket is a valuable item to own, fulfilling as it does both a fully functional purpose with all the correct equipment in a specially designed container and completion of your outfit with a certain dash and attention to detail that will certainly impress others.

SPORTS TOILETRIES

There are a variety of sporting occasions when a toiletry bag is a vital accessory for a gentleman's well-being as well as his grooming. At the gym, it is essential to freshen up after strenuous exercise, but after many sporting activities it makes a huge difference to be able to wash your hair, apply fresh deodorant, and clean your teeth. A small neat bag, preferably in a tough sporty nylon to team with your sports bag and containing only the essentials, is a truly functional accessory. Depending on the sporting activity, it is also an excellent place to store support bandages, muscle strain applications, or simply band-aids to cover minor cuts and scratches.

Tip *Sweaty and disheveled is only manly in the movies. In real life, you just look hot and bothered—always shower and change your clothes after the game.*

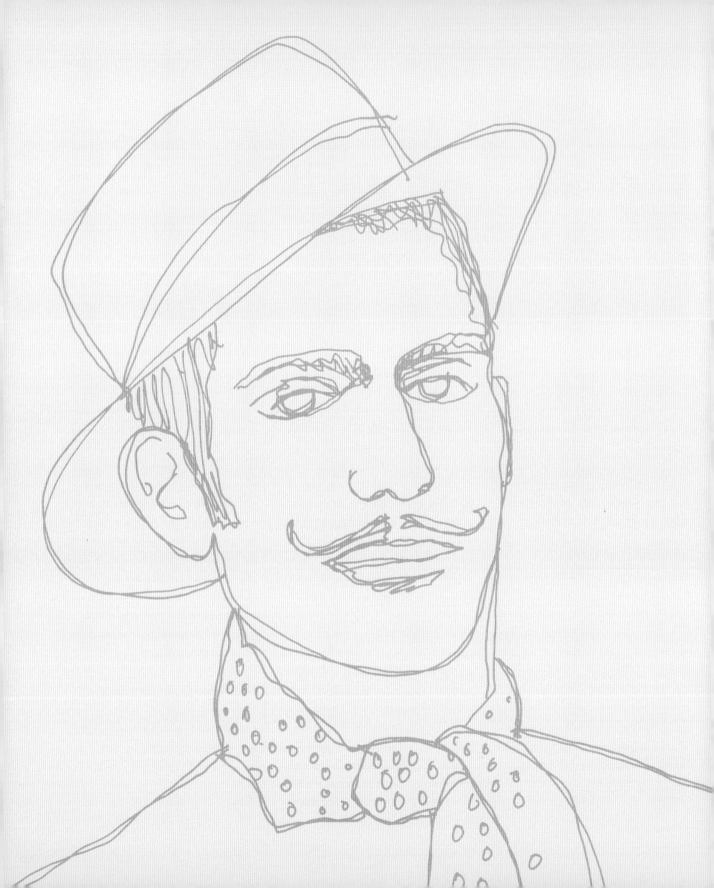

"The designers who would leave their mark on the twenty-first century ... are not all Belgian, but they do all work in Antwerp or Brussels, which is why they are often classified as Belgian."

VEERLE WINDELS, FASHION JOURNALIST

CREATIVE DRESSING SUITS

For many men the suit is less of a statement and more of a straitjacket. Whether because of profession or personality, some feel a need to express more through their clothes than the conventional suit can. Fashion strives to move even classic items into new realms of creativity, and there are many designers who achieve this with excellent results. Creative dressing is an option for those who have either the attitude or the profession to wear a less-than-classic interpretation of the suit.

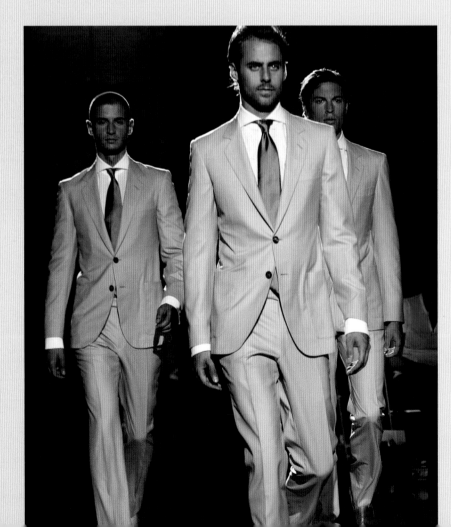

If you are a creative dresser, your suit may differ in one of several areas, but you must avoid too many conflicting design elements. Although the key players in this arena are expert at avoiding overstatement, there are catwalk pieces and attention grabbers that are worn for the press or purchased to dress store windows to cause controversy rather than generate sales; so beware.

Never buy a suit that you plan to wear over a period of time yet is so distinctive that it becomes over familiar after being worn only two or three times. Never, ever, buy a suit with every design element overworked. The suit may be a fresh silhouette, have interesting details, or be made of an unconventional fabric, but never all three at the same time, if you wish to avoid ridicule.

Left: *The flash of white cuff and shirt front and the gray tie combined with a neutral suit demonstrate how detail and balance can make a stylish statement.*

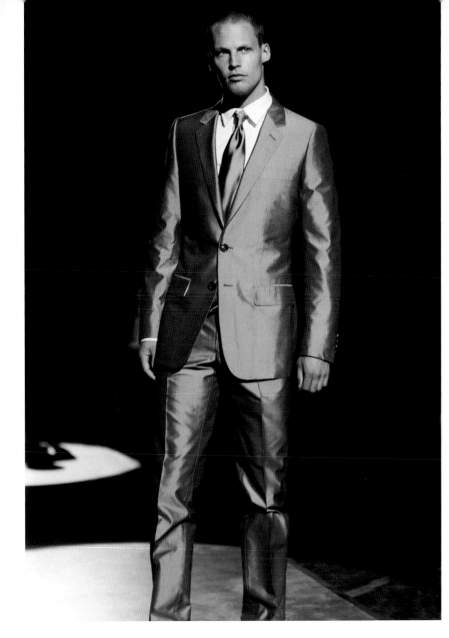

DETAIL

Designers have a great many possibilities to play with even on a classic suit: buttons and fastenings, pockets and pocket details, stitching and embroidery, braid and ribbon, and other decorative details. Other details may include hidden design features such as cuff lining, braided edge to the lining, contrast under collar, or details hidden under pocket flaps.

FABRIC

The fabric may have a unique weave or surface construction, it may have a specialized color, or it may be a classic fabric used in a distinctive or unusual way. Many designer fabrics are less durable and harder to care for than conventional suiting, so you should check the fiber content and cleaning advice carefully before purchase. As with all suit fabrics, try on the complete outfit and stand well back from the mirror to gauge the total effect. It may be the look of the moment and it may be a hot designer name, but that does not mean it is perfect for your wardrobe, proportions, coloring, business, or lifestyle.

SILHOUETTE

The basic structure of your creative suit may differ from the norm with extremes of both make and proportion, thus altering the silhouette of the suit. Longer or shorter and wider or narrower are the key elements in changing the design. A jacket shorter than the current convention is one possibility, or much longer, edging toward a tailcoat, another variation. Either much slimmer cut or softly oversized also offer a challenge to the suit buyer. The construction may be underpinned differently from the classic suit, with padded shoulders, external stitching, or other modifications.

Tip Details are often strong on creative suits, so examine them carefully as you go through the store.

Tip Designer suits often still work after their season at the cutting edge, so check the sale racks for something stylish.

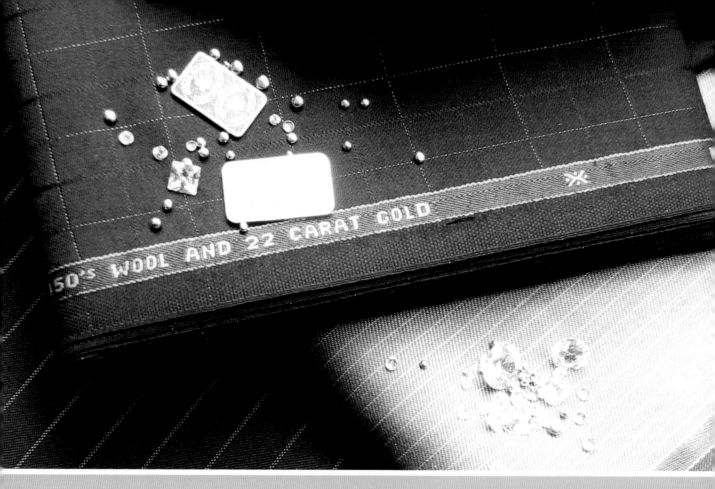

PATTERN & JACKETS

Many men who are generally conservative and classic in their dress can make a serious sartorial faux pas when it comes to pattern—an elaborate fancy sweater, a wild holiday shirt, or a silly novelty vest; however, pattern does have a role to play within any gentleman's wardrobe, especially if he is a creative dresser. Color and fabric can also lead some gentlemen astray into unsuitable tricks with fashion that do not fit in with either their style or their business. Avoid these disasters by using your general color sense and style as a starting point and building from this area of success. For example, if you wear a great deal of mid-toned gray you can add gray-based textural fabrics, gray with black and white, and patterns in soft tones that have a gray tint to them such as rose-gray, blue-gray, or green-gray.

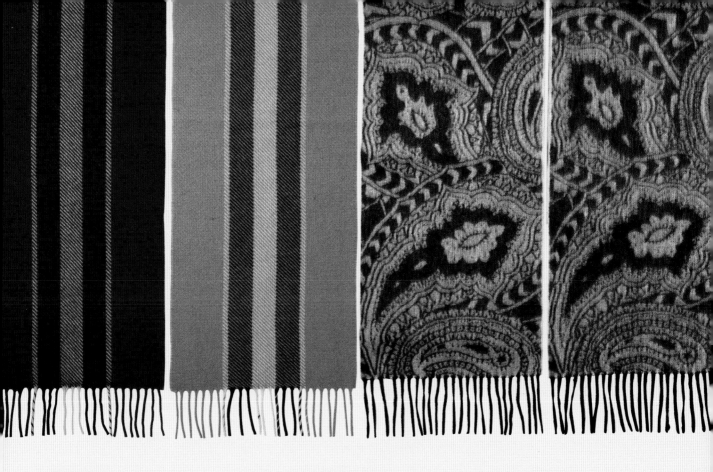

ACCESSORIES

Ties, vests, and scarves can all introduce pattern in a subtle but creative way into the gentleman's attire. This may include statement fabrics and colors as well as the pattern, but in proportion to the suit or outfit, the accessories should not overpower, or the total look will overwhelm. Bold scarves tucked into the neck of a suit or coat can create a slightly dandy image without going too far, and since they are generally removed and laid aside after the initial statement, allow for self-expression. Vests, like ties, are a flash at the neck rather than a full-length statement. Designer scarves have gained a greater acceptance for men in recent years, and if you explore clever fabrics, bold colors, or interesting surface treatments, you will discover

how much they may add to an outfit. Surprisingly, there are scarves for all seasons, including summer, when they can be very practical in case of sudden weather changes.

JACKETS

Jackets in patterns are available in a wide range of styles and options. It might be a creative variation on the classic—a pinstripe on velvet, or a classic jacket with a decorative lining that will only be glimpsed. Creative dressers will also look at the special jacket that makes a statement, yet is still classic-based. Longer jackets with a hint of tails have gone in and out of fashion. The fabric may be conservative and the cut vintage-inspired, but the shape makes a strong statement and, for many men, a flattering silhouette.

If you are in good shape, slim cut is always a great option. Conversely, if you are larger, do not imagine that an oversize garment will flatter; it should reflect ease and proportion, along with length, which is often a strong contributor to the effectiveness of the flattering qualities of the garment if you are shorter than average. Above all, it is fabric that can make the statement in a jacket, often changing a classic cut into a creative garment, so when shopping, look carefully at the special or one-of-a-kind jacket as a statement in your wardrobe.

Tip *Always bear in mind your body mass for pattern: if you are small-boned, choose a smaller pattern; if you have a solid frame, you can go bolder.*

VESTS

Vests are surprisingly subject to the whims of fashion. There are single-breasted and Regency-inspired double-breasted styles; the neck may be V-shape or rounded. Whatever the style, all require a certain panache to wear, which is one of the reasons why the vest is often a formal item for the gentleman of today. Remember that a tight-buttoned vest gives prominence to the stomach and does not act as a corset.

SUIT VESTS The three-piece suit is a concept that appeals to certain gentlemen. The vest should be absolutely classic in concept and in complete harmony with the style of the suit. The vest should have a discreet tonal lining for the back with an adjustable half-belt that is never left unfastened. If the jacket is kept buttoned, an unfastened belt leaves an unsightly lump at the back and when the jacket is removed in the heat of business it looks untidy and unprofessional dangling from the back of the vest.

Tip *Think of the colors and styles you wear most often when looking at tones or fabrics for a vest.*

NOVELTY VESTS As with all novelty items, the answer is always emphatically, "No." Christmas vests with reindeer and Santas tumbling across them, Valentine vests with bright pink hearts scattered everywhere—these and others like them should be avoided at all costs. These styles are often badly cut and made of cheap synthetic fabrics, thus also declaring their novelty factor in their cheapness. They are basically saying, "To be worn only once and laughed at."

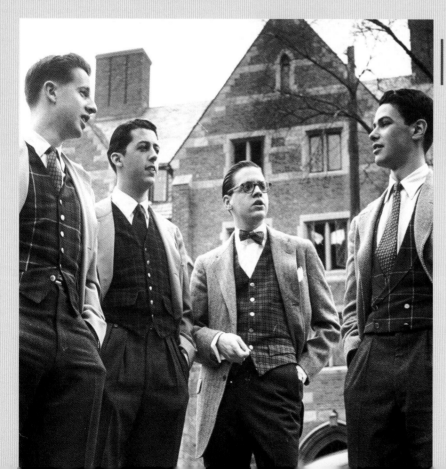

Left: *Little has changed with the classic vest in over a hundred years.*

rough, scratchy, abrasive brocades. The back of the vest may be of brocade or satin; if satin, it should either be matching or a luxury color such as ivory, rose pink, pale lemon, or ice blue. Buttons should be very discreet since the fabric is doing the work of dazzling the observer.

Tip Do not ignore vests; they can serve as color or fabric accents in your wardrobe.

VELVET The contrast between the matte blackness of a tuxedo or other evening suit and the rich texture of velvet is a timeless style statement. The best velvet vests are from designers who use top-quality fabrics and jewel-like buttons. Black is best, but, as with brocade, a rich almost-black shade is an option: aubergine, forest green, bitter chocolate, or black shot with lacquer red.

COUNTRY SQUIRE Moleskin, wool plush, suede, and tapestry are all possible fabrics for vests with a bohemian quality to them. In rustic colors such as corn, peat, or slate, they may appear classic and country in feel, especially if worn with tweeds and corduroys; in more adventurous tones of color they veer toward statement dressing. Dense floral colors and even Liberty print-style vests add a witty punctuation to conventional clothing.

BROCADE Weddings and some dinner events suit a decorative vest fabric, especially a fabric with shimmer and richness to show up under candlelight or festive lighting. Rich dark colors such as plum, fir green, pewter, or Bordeaux work well. With a pale gray or lightweight suit, go for tonal shades such as café au lait, silver gray or lavender. Make sure the fabric is as expensive as you can manage and has a soft touch. Avoid

CREATIVE GROOMING

Although a touch of creativity, or even eccentricity, rarely requires advice, there may be elements of creative style that you admire. You may wish to consider adapting them to your business or life, but wonder about their application.

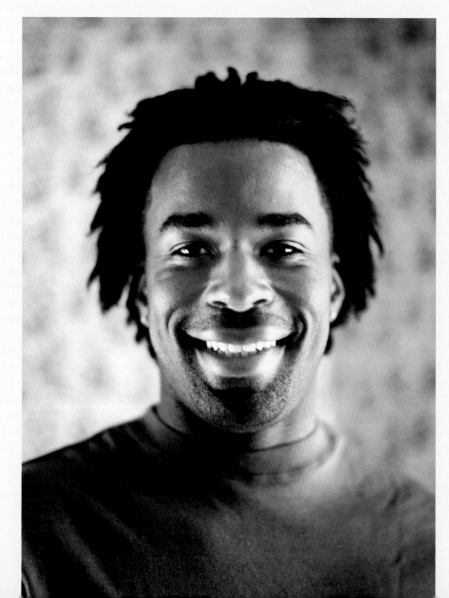

Left: *Although creative, this hair and beard combination is not overstated.*

HAIR & FACIAL HAIR

Extremes of statement with wild hairstyles shaved into weird shapes, plaited into bizarre confections, or simply allowed to grow free can be great conversation starters, but they will rarely mark you out as smart, well-styled, or as a candidate for possible promotion to senior management. Likewise, facial hair that resembles nothing so much as eighteenth-century garden topiary will help you to stand out in the crowd. On the other hand, if you have hair which has a special character and yet still looks slick, groomed, and stylish, or you suit a Vandyke goatee (a neat chin beard shaped into a point) then by all means adopt it. The key points here are to ensure that it will enhance and suit your appearance, that you have the panache and air to carry it off, and that the style adopted is suitable for your work environment. As ever, the care, cleanliness, and maintenance of any style is paramount.

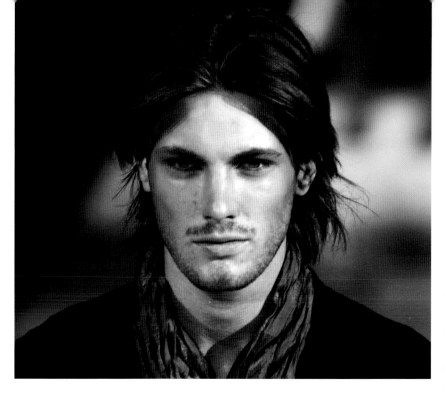

Left: Stylish long hair and stubble is here set off by a creatively twisted scarf.

SHOES

If classic shoes seem dull and you wish to make your footwear more creative, bear in mind some key factors. Quality is first; do not buy cheap fashion-style footwear that will scuff and split within weeks; even if you wish to go for something more creative, continue to buy good footwear. Second, make certain that your shoes match the rest of your wardrobe and style; a strictly conventional and classic suit with a stand-out designer shoe may look odd. Finally, check the style publications and stores before making a purchase that may either be out of date before you wear it or spends most of its life languishing in the dark recesses of your closet. If you want to make a statement with footwear, go for the best of top-level shoemakers; this will ensure that the shoes you buy will not only last and repair well, but will also have been created with the discerning client in mind, not just for instant fashion effect.

ACCESSORIES & DETAILS

Tinted eyewear throughout the year, huge encompassing wrap scarves, or bizarrely designed messenger bags are all elements of creative dressing that can look dashing; however, they may also make you look affected, stupid, or as if trying too hard. Only you will know, when you try any of the more creative twists, which ones work to empower you and make you feel special, and which ones make you feel self-conscious and nervous.

Tip *Watch creative television programs to get an idea of what stylists are selecting for celebrities and actors.*

There is a huge selection of creative accessories to choose from, so, whether buying a simple neck chain or a wonderful ankle-length coat, be sure you are going to get your money's worth from the purchase. Often hidden or subtle design statements

can be as creative as overstatement. The lining and the facing (the backing fabric to collars and cuffs) are great areas to introduce exotic, floral, or colored fabrics: perhaps a red under-collar to a navy Crombie coat, or a floral lining to a spring suit. A simple or classic jacket can be transformed by a row of special buttons on the cuff or some discreet, colored top stitching. Style publications will demonstrate the newest methods of finish that designers are exploring. Since the 1990s, deconstruction has been a constant creative element for many designers; this often involves finish and edge treatments for tailoring. Military detailing is another constant influence, even on classic clothing; in fact, military is itself classic, but it is the application to non-military clothing that shows creativity. Buttoning, braiding, and pocket details are all part of this creative style, yet are often low-key and of the finest quality, rather than overstated.

Tip *Visit stores that are both cutting-edge and creative to see what they have on the racks; this will give you an overview of the commonalities of detail, color, and fabric for creative style.*

THE WORLD OF MENSWEAR DESIGNERS

There are many men who work in professions where a more creative attitude toward dress is not only tolerated, it is expected as part of the presentation. Generally speaking, it is assumed that if you are in the creative industries you will be more focused on this type of dressing. You will not only know where to purchase designer garments but what to buy, how to wear it, and who the hot new names are. Other men shy away from this area of style and often feel it is irrelevant to them. Curiosity is an excellent stimulus for style and is to be encouraged. Experimental and directional designers influence future trends, so instead of ignoring them, discover who they are, what they do, why they are important to certain people, and if there are things you can learn or take away to use and adapt for your own wardrobe style.

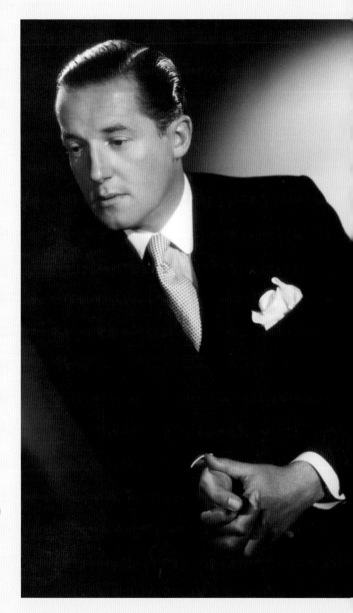

CREATIVE DRESSING

GLOBAL MENSWEAR
FASHION DESIGNERS

If France is traditionally the home of the best of fashion design for women, then London and Italy have the crown for menswear. Savile Row custom tailoring and Giorgio Armani in Italy are possibly the two most important names that a gentleman should be aware of if asked about style. In the last twenty years or so, there have been other shifts in the fashion element of menswear; even the formal and classic. Japanese designers like Yohji Yamamoto and Rei Kawakubo, along with Belgian designers such as Raf Simons and Martin Margiela, have proved their staying power within the business and have a solid customer base globally for their interpretations of menswear garments from the suit to the shoe. Their strongly individual view of menswear and the statement that it makes about the wearer is not for everybody, but do not instantly dismiss their complete output. Although catwalk items, and much of what they do, may not be for you, it is worth investigating their clothes when the opportunity arises. Perhaps try some things on, not only to discover and understand what they do, but also for the occasional item that will work within your wardrobe and add a zest to your style. Like seasoning in food, a dash of fashion may save you from blandness and lack of presence. You do not have to buy a top-to-toe look, but a simple but special white shirt, a terrific scarf, or perhaps a great designer wallet will add panache to your wardrobe.

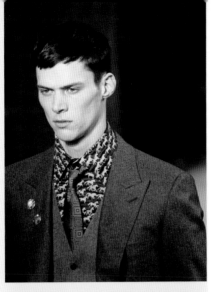

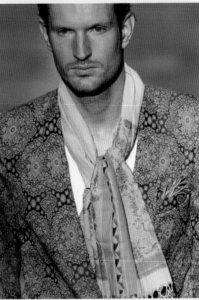

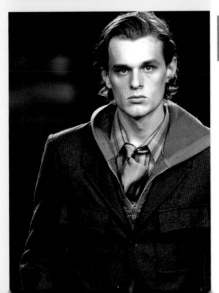

LOCAL DESIGNERS

Every designer bases his collections on the experience of his surrounding core customers: the gentlemen who live with the same climate, the same traditions, and the same heritage as himself. Calvin Klein and Ralph Lauren have established their core customer in America because they understand exactly who these men are. New-generation designers and local tailors will follow in their footsteps and develop clothing for a man that reflects the world they live in. New names are there to be investigated and tried out, new names are to be supported, and local talent starting out should be promoted by the local community. This is about learning and communicating about men's clothing. If you wish to achieve success in both your professional and private life, it is important in today's visually aware society to devote adequate time and effort to dressing. Creative dressing may be a small part of your wardrobe and your life, but can be dangerous to ignore completely from the point of personal style development.

Tip When considering international creative clothing, think of the countries you respond to most readily, then investigate their designers.

Left: *The bold-cut jacket collar and classic vest are set off by the patterned shirt (top); a patterned jacket and scarf work because they are tonal in color and compatible in scale (center); mixing casual with formal and keeping the color complementary creates a chic, understated look (bottom).*

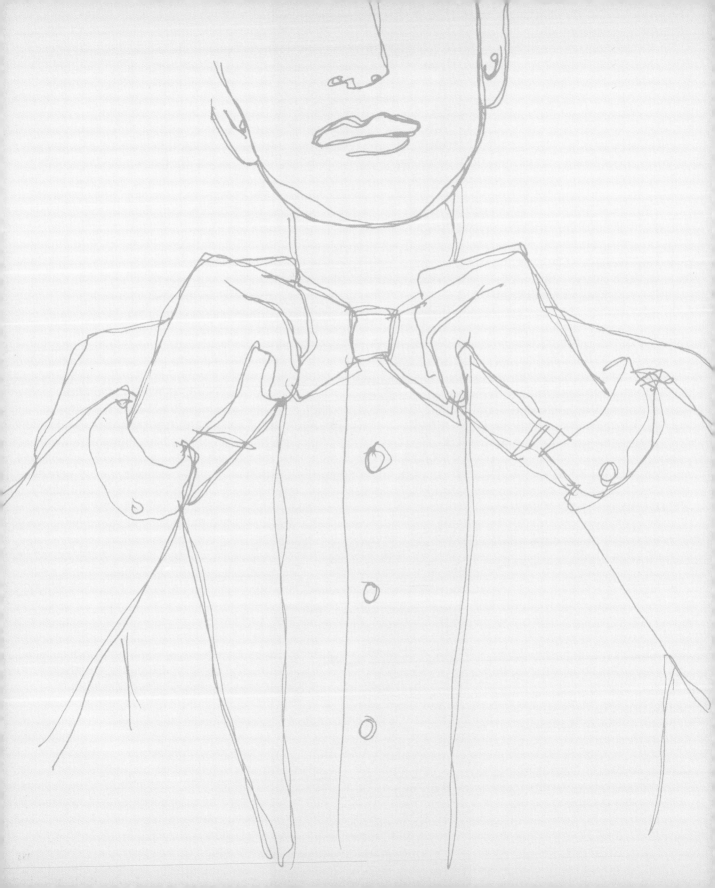

"Until the 1970s nobody
really thought about what
men wore to the Oscars. The
requisite tuxedo provided the
appropriate background for
the ladies in their dramatic
finery. The biggest choice was
whether to wear a boutonniere
or a pocket square."

*PATTY FOX, ACADEMY AWARDS
FASHION COORDINATOR*

THE TUXEDO

The tuxedo, or dinner suit, is designed both as a graphic statement for the gentleman and as a superb foil for the woman, whatever she may choose to wear. The basic style has changed little in the past 100 years, since like any great classic all it ever needs is modifying and updating from time to time. This does mean that a dinner suit cannot be worn indefinitely since styles do change, and over the seasons fashion influences the silhouette, number of buttons, and lapel width.

SUITS Evening suits should be black or a navy blue so dark it appears black; the suit should also be in a medium-weight fabric. Take a corner of the suit fabric in your hand and crumple it up; if it springs back to shape quickly, this is a sign that over a long evening seated your suit will not look crumpled when you stand up. The lapels of the suit can be in satin or silk; the silk may be ribbed or plain, and the satin should have a subtle sheen but not look highly polished. Buttons are best plain or with a very discreet designer motif to them. The trouser shape will follow the same rules as formalwear trousers, as will the number of buttons on the jacket. (*See The Basics of Fitting a Suit, p. 43*) The satin stripe down the side of the trousers is optional, as are

satin cuffs, pocket flaps, or buttons. It is best to avoid too many matching details; otherwise, just as when a woman wears a fussy dress, the attire will be noticed more than the wearer. When buying your tuxedo, it is advisable to consider the type of functions you will wear it at during the coming months—dinners, cocktails, charity events, theater gala, making a speech, receiving an award, hosting an event, and so on. This will help in your decision regarding both style and expenditure. Consider whether you are likely to be the center of attention or host and need to make a statement with your suit, or whether you will be merely part of a crowd and need only wear something plain and classic. At today's more relaxed formal

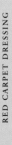

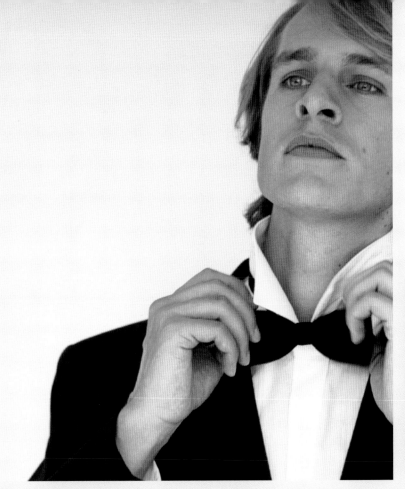

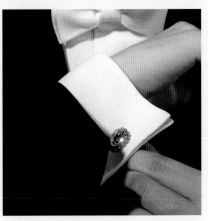

Left and below: The details of classic tuxedo dressing count for a lot in the style stakes.

occasions, the tuxedo jacket may be teamed with a white shirt and jeans for a new mix; remember that the jacket should still be of the top quality and design and the jeans of the moment—this is not an excuse to become scruffy, but to make an alternative style statement.

Tip Never, ever, rent a dinner suit. That is all there is to be said. Ever.

JACKETS Black velvet jackets have become a classic option for evening events, and they are also suitable in color. Choose a dark color for several reasons: it will be less memorable on repeated wearings than too strong or bright a color; it will not clash with anything your partner may wear;

and it can be worn with a classic black trouser, thus avoiding extra expense and shoe problems. The shape should follow the correct style for your body shape and subtly reflect fashion in the matter of lapel shape and details.

INVESTITURES, EMBASSY FUNCTIONS, OR WEDDINGS

Although there are still some very grand occasions and events, generally dressing within one's lifestyle, social milieu, and income bracket means that if you are invited to such a level of formal event, you should carefully check to ascertain the level of grandeur. As an example, the role of the tailcoat has diminished in recent years, and even the conductor of a classical symphony

orchestra will have hunted for alternative modern variations. If the occasion should arise for the wearing of either a tailcoat or full-morning dress it is highly advisable to seek expert opinion on what is acceptable for the specific occasion. Depending on the level of your professional standing and the corresponding social life, it is unlikely that either of these versions of evening dress will be essential basics within your wardrobe.

Tip If you are attending a grand formal event, it is an excellent idea to check the titles and mode of address of dignitaries or royalty, thus avoiding any social faux pas.

RED CARPET SHIRTS

Although evening dress is a limited element in most men's wardrobes, there is a dazzling array of possibilities within evening shirts.

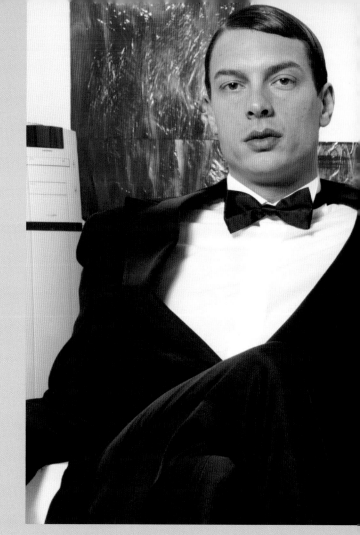

WING COLLARS The wing-collared shirt is not always in fashion, and it has certain elements that are difficult; for example, the way the points lie on the collar may be uneven; if the bow tie is not tied straight around the neck the whole collar appears to be uneven; the depth of the collar stand may not be the fashion of the times. The worst is a collar of one size teamed with a ready-made bow tie of another, which either then squeezes the neck or floats around it. All these problems must be solved if the wing-collared shirt is to be successful when worn.

CLASSIC COLLARS Although classic might imply boring and conventional, what is meant here is appropriate and surprisingly versatile: it is the plain collar. The plain collar is easy to manage. It may be cutaway, high-necked, or pointed, but it is based on the classic shirt collar rather than evening dress and it is the addition of tuxedo, bow tie, and styling details that move its use to evening.

Tip An evening shirt should be dazzling white, crisp, and fresh; if in doubt, buy a new shirt.

RUFFLES A single dramatic flourish or several small-scale ruffles? Applied all the way down the shirt or only on a bib front? All of the options mentioned have a different event application and so a man may have several evening shirts to enable him to select the most appropriate. A soft white cotton shirt with several rows of small ruffles has a slightly informal, cowboy or country-and-western style to it, while a shirt with a bigger stiff collar and a single bold ruffle hints at Regency style and is therefore grander.

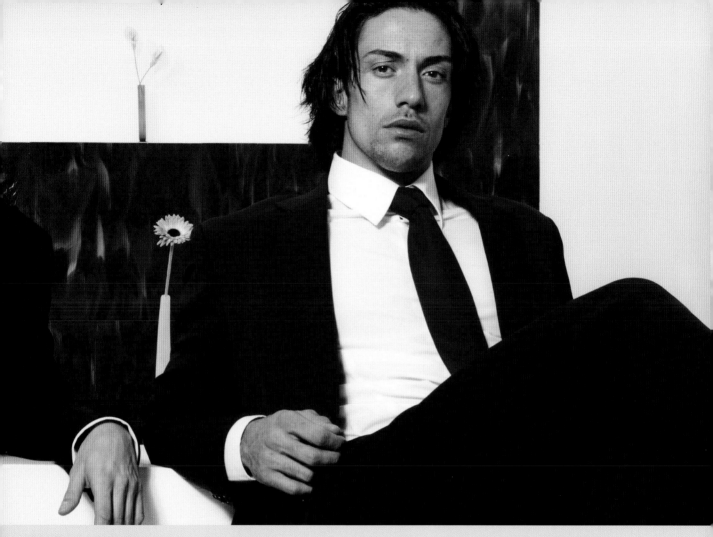

Above: *Black tie variations. Both gentlemen are sticking to the rules and are appropriately attired, but are displaying different interpretations of red carpet dressing.*

TUXEDO SHIRTS The bib-effect front on a tuxedo shirt is designed so that no decoration on the shirt front will interfere with the line of a dress vest. (Note: A dress vest is usually white with a cutaway back fastened with a strap and buckle.) Today this design is still used without the waistcoat. Tucked or pleated fabric is the classic style but sometimes a different fabric is used, such as piqué

Tip *If you wear evening dress infrequently, try your shirt on a few days before an event to make sure it still fits.*

FRENCH CUFFS These are important for an evening shirt since the sharp contrast of the white with the black suit or tuxedo is quite dramatic; accessorized with great cufflinks, the classic style is unbeatable.

COLOR White is obviously the preferred choice with its crisp contrast to black, and it avoids clashing with any color your partner may choose. The colored dinner shirt is also an option, whether ruffled, pleated, or plain. Retro pastel shades, possibly even a vintage shirt, can make a real style statement, as can a totally

unexpected color such as orange or lime. The one consideration is how many times you may wear such statement items; you will not want to be seen by the same people in the same shirt every time. Black shirts have been a fashion in recent seasons, followed by dark tones, usually worn with a matching silk tie, but this is as likely to become outdated and vulgar as any fashion whim. White is not only smarter and more flattering, it is more versatile. You can look stylish without a tie, but for a more creative formal occasion, add a patterned tie or bow tie in satin, velvet, or brocade.

RED CARPET ACCESSORIES

The final touches given to any red carpet outfit can be a major pleasure. Gentlemen rarely get the chance to indulge in the more extravagant elements within the style repertoire, but red carpet dressing gives the opportunity to go just a little bit further without running the risk of overstatement. Cufflinks, watches, scarves, the lining of the tuxedo, all add that discreet "luxe" that shimmers in the night light.

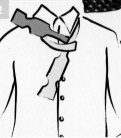

TIES & BOWTIES It is permissible nowadays to wear a tie for evening events, but the tie should reflect current fashions in color, width, and fabric. Black on black and white on white have been popular for some years, but white on black runs the danger of making you look like a retro gangster, so be careful.

A bow tie should always be made of the best possible quality heavy silk. Before purchasing your tie, check out what the style leaders are wearing for black tie events for an update on size of the bow, because this shifts subtly over the years. In the 70s, bowties were huge and often velvet, in the 80s, narrow and neat in satin, and at present matte fabrics with solid but not oversized bows are in fashion.

Your bowtie should never, ever, under any circumstances whatsoever, be ready-made. You must practice tying the knot, or find out if your partner can help.

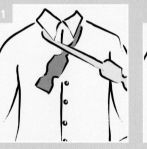

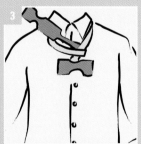

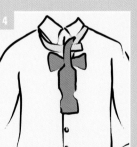

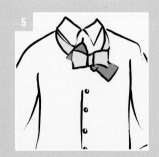

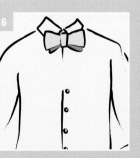

1. Cross the tie over.
2. Loop the other half through.
3. Fold one half of the bow.
4. Fold second bow half and loop through.
5. Slip the half bow through the bow center.
6. Hold both halves of the bow and tighten.

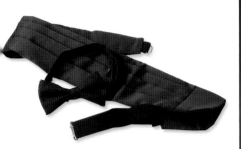

CUMMERBUNDS The idea of a corset-like structure around your waist for the evening may not appeal, but there are times when the cummerbund is a true style statement. The shape may be the classic pleated satin style with a strap and buckle fastening at the back, or it may be a flat-cut designer version with small buttons; either way, the addition of this accessory is to be considered carefully. Danger areas include slipping, undue stomach emphasis, and simply being out of fashion or overdressed. As with all novelty items, cummerbunds in amusing prints are to be avoided, especially if they match the bow tie and handkerchief.

Tip *Take new items out of their packaging twenty-four hours before the event to allow the creases to drop out.*

CUFFLINKS should be classic and may include subtle sparkle with an antique flavor, but flashy gems are simply vulgar. If you wear a shirt with studs, these may also contain enamel or sparkle but again, words such as heritage, vintage, and heirloom are the best to direct your style.

BOUTONNIERES In recent seasons we have seen a return in the fashion for a flower on a gentleman's lapel. A fresh flower, appearing to be picked from your own garden and nonchalantly pinned on, can be charming at a garden party, regatta, or some such event.

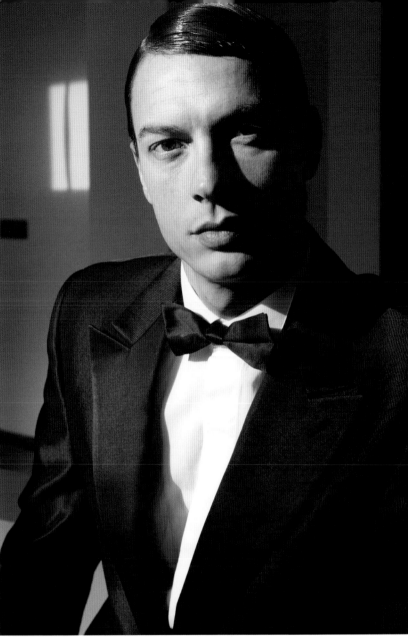

Above: Bow ties have varied enormously in size over the years; shown here is a classic, smaller, neat bow, worn with a low-buttoning jacket. *Above left:* Because the black silk cummerbund has a timeless elegance, it may be stored until the right evening event comes along.

SCARVES There is really only one scarf to be worn in the evening: a white silk scarf in the classic style, that is, an oblong, with a knotted fringe at each end. The fabric should be expensive and soft in a chalk-white or pale ivory. Never buy a cheap evening scarf in stiff, optical white fabric.

Note *A miniature version of a medal or award, such as the Légion d'Honneur, can also be worn on the lapel. Likewise, a discreet diamond pin, if you have the élan to carry it off.*

FOOTWEAR AND GROOMING FOR RED CARPET DRESSING

The aim of a gentleman on a special or gala night is to appear polished and debonair. A visit to the hairdresser or manicurist, extra time in the bathroom, all add to the sense of the occasion. Take your time to go through your routine, accompanied, perhaps, by a glass of champagne to get you in the mood.

SHOES Evening shoes should be of light construction since they are not worn for practical reasons. Classic styles–whether lace up, slip on, or boot–are best. They should be black, obviously, but highly polished or even patent leather indicates that the shoes are not everyday but reserved for special occasions. Another evening shoe option is what are termed evening pumps or dancing shoes; these are based on Regency men's shoes and are almost like a slipper, with a small low heel, and are often decorated with a flat grosgrain bow on the front. This type of shoe should always be worn with a thin silk sock and, since the shoe is lower-cut at the front, the sock will be clearly visible.

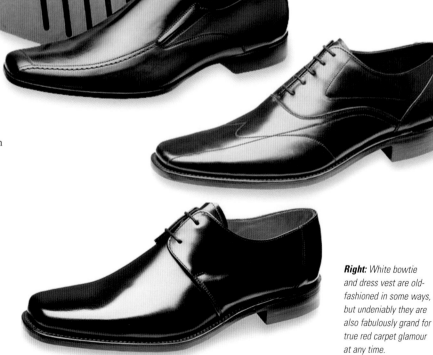

Right: Beautifully polished shoes in soft leather complement a classic dinner suit.

Right: White bowtie and dress vest are old-fashioned in some ways, but undeniably they are also fabulously grand for true red carpet glamour at any time.

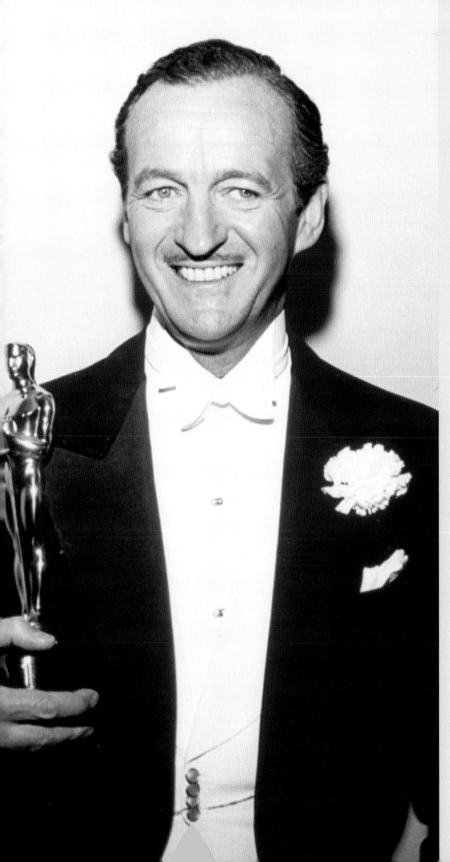

RED CARPET GROOMING A special occasion calls for special treatment, and taking the time to visit your hairdresser, go for a massage, and have a facial scrub will all add to your confidence. Next to impeccable white cuffs with the discreet glimmer of vintage gold cufflinks, a well-manicured hand is essential. At formal events you will make more of an entrance than simply arriving, and the added grooming time of face, hands, hair, and body will augment your well-being as you arrive. Whatever your hairstyle, make certain your hair is spotlessly clean, groomed, and styled; remember, there are likely to be photographs taken, and a slapdash attitude for the finer details will be recorded forever as a reminder of your lack of planning and care.

It is often to be noted that many male celebrities take the step of styling their hair into classic vintage Hollywood style for red carpet events. Slicked back or side-parted hair may look too contrived for everyday choice, but with a dinner jacket and under flashbulbs it can transform the way you feel and look.

If you are escorting a woman in cocktail or evening dress, one of the greatest compliments you can pay her is to provide the perfect partner in sartorial polish to her own efforts. The silver screen has over the years provided some great and timeless style pointers, and these can inspire you from the hairstyles down in top-to-toe classic style for any gentleman.

FOOTWEAR AND GROOMING FOR RED CARPET DRESSING

143

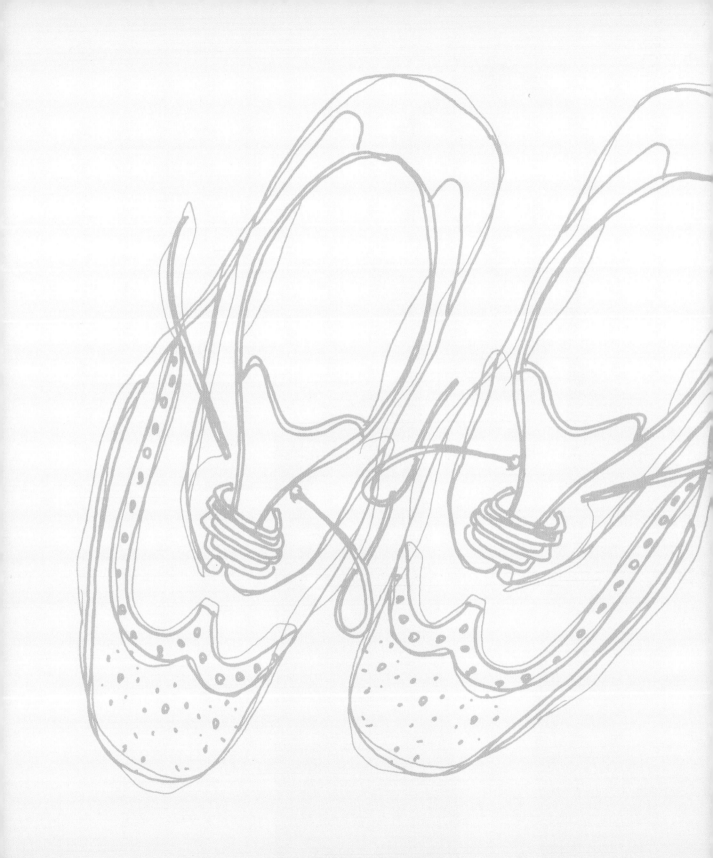

"Tiffany design is cool, direct, plainspoken as it appeals to the senses. Like all good Americans, it is economical in its means."

JOHN LORING, TIFFANY & CO. DESIGN DIRECTOR

HATS

Any accessories a gentleman adds to his wardrobe should address at least one of the following questions: Does it enhance my overall style statement? Is it adding practicality? Will I wear it often enough to justify the purchase? These questions are especially relevant to hats and headgear in general.

BERET The beret is a traditional French felt hat from Brittany, with no details except a small "stalk" on the top where the felt shape is finished. The beret evokes the French countryside, traditional onion sellers, or French painters such as Monet. If you feel it suits you, it is definitely a classic, but its associations may elicit laughter rather than admiration from your companions.

BEANIE The beanie is virtually any small pull-on hat in fleece, jersey, or knit fabric. The beanie may be worn at a variety of angles and rolled to sit on the back of the head or pulled right down over the ears. Beanies come in every color and pattern possible and it is a personal matter as to which suits your lifestyle and coloring.

Tip A hat frames your face, so its color is important. If you are blond, a beige hat could make you look bald; if you have a ruddy complexion, a red hat could make you resemble a tomato.

FEDORA A soft, wide-brimmed hat style that has a dented crown, introduced in 1881, the fedora is associated with gangsters and retro style and makes a bold style statement. Unless you are certain you can carry it off with panache, and it is appropriate to your lifestyle and business, then it is best left to others. If you do purchase a fedora it should be made from top quality felt in a dark classic shade such as black or navy with a firm ribbon band around the crown.

TRILBY A classic hat with a dented crown and a medium-width rolled brim, the Trilby is named after the George du Maurier book of the same name and first became popular in the 1890s. Although a stylish hat to wear, its heyday was during the Hollywood

Left: The classic bowler hat may be aging on a more mature man, but has an appealing respect for tradition on someone younger.

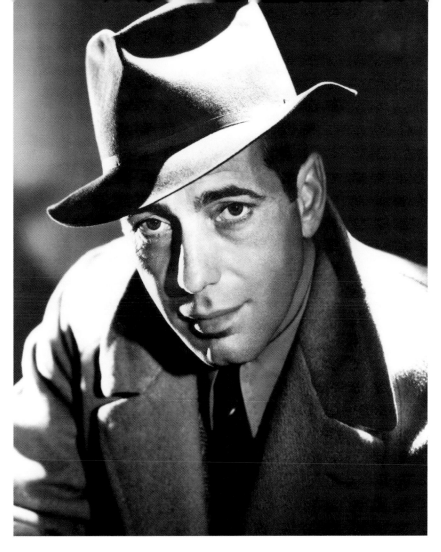

years of the 30s and 40s; thus, like so many seemingly classic hat styles, it requires a degree of confidence to pull it off effectively as a look.

BOWLER HAT Even in London, where this most traditional of British hats was first made by Bowler the Feltmaker in the 1840s, the bowler hat has long been a symbol of the businessman. However, this style has rapidly diminished in contemporary society. The hat is made of hard felt and shaped with a domed crown and a small brim with a plain ribbon around the crown. Since this is such a traditional, indeed old-fashioned style, it is not an easy one to make work today.

STETSON The classic cowboy or Western hat of choice, this is not a hat to wear for fashion. It is a style statement and should only be worn if you have the lifestyle and panache to carry it off. The only other time to wear a Stetson is if you are at a Village People reunion party or a costume ball.

CAP The classic cap as worn by the British country gentleman is a great practical headwear style that comes in a terrific range of colors and fabrics from tweed and corduroy to synthetics, nylons, and sporty cottons. The crown part of the cap may be fuller in cut, even with panels, than the traditional "flat" cap, but the general structure and style is the same. The cap may be worn at various angles and is versatile enough to suit styles from dark formal business attire to a fun nightclub look.

BASEBALL CAP Practical, classic, and masculine—what could possibly go wrong with a baseball cap? Make absolutely sure the cap is a good fit and perched neither on top of your head nor over your ears. Be certain that any logo, motif, or initials on the hat are ones you wish to promote. Finally, does it work with the rest of your outfit and, classic though it may be, does its style suit you? Not every man looks good in a baseball cap, and teamed with more formal styles it can just look plain silly.

TOP HAT The grandest and most formal hat still used in the gentleman's wardrobe, the top hat is a Victorian style that has endured through the centuries. It is generally only worn today for weddings, funerals, some formal race meetings, and state occasions. For most men it will be a question of renting such a hat, since there is little likelihood of needing one regularly.

Tip Always wear a hat with absolute confidence, or it simply won't work for you.

HATS

LEATHER GOODS

A black wallet for town, a brown one for the country; a sleek, polished black-leather belt for the city and a tooled brown-hide one for a rural weekend. The leather goods that complete your outfit can make a surprisingly strong statement. These are not the follies of fashion but the necessities of a gentleman's everyday existence.

WALLET A gentleman's wallet can speak volumes about his style and attention to detail. The first prerequisite is that it should be large enough to contain the essential cash and credit cards. This is the purpose for which a wallet is intended. Avoid using it for dog-eared receipts, old business cards, a photograph of the family pet, and a ticket stub from the movies six months ago; in other words, at the end of each day sort out your wallet and transfer items either to the trashcan or the filing cabinet. Your wallet should be of a suitable size to fit into a document case or possibly an inside jacket pocket. However, remember that a large or overfilled wallet forced into a snug-fitting jacket will distort the line of the garment and in time ruin the fabric. All classic wallets come in leather of a variety of types from plain to exotic animal or reptile skins. It is common sense to have several wallet styles: a small flat one for weekend shopping, a large sturdy one for business, a waterproof one for vacationing, and even a sports-style wallet to use at the gym, sports club, or during sporting activities.

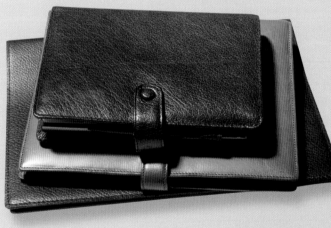

Left: *It is advisable to have a selection of wallets in different styles, fabrics, and colors; all leather goods should be the best quality you can afford.*

CARD HOLDERS If you are in business and use a business card, it is a good idea to purchase an appropriate card container. This might be metal or leather and may also be used to place cards given to you for safekeeping. In some countries, the culture demands that business cards be exchanged at all meetings, so check on this before travel. You may also be able to arrange in advance for cards with your name and details printed in the language of the country.

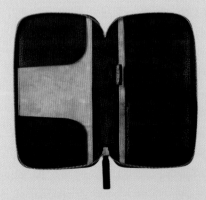

Above: *Small leather goods should be kept in tip-top condition. Worn and scruffy items should be replaced.*

BELTS A belt is a functional item, therefore it should fit your waist and the notch for the buckle prong to pass through should be comfortable. Never wear a belt which either sits below your stomach or forces all the fabric to bulge either side, making you resemble an overstuffed sausage. The variety of belts available may lead to confusion and there are some real sartorial pitfalls waiting for the unwary with widths and buckle styles.

The general rule is that for business, town, and the suit, the belt should be approximately one- to one-and-a half inches in width, plain leather, with a small neat buckle, which should be in harmony with other metal in your wardrobe. So, if you have a silver watch strap and cufflinks and a generally cool-colored wardrobe, the belt buckles should be silver. Fancy buckles are distinctly unwise for business and the Western-style buckle, the designer logo belt, or a belt made in heavily tooled leather should remain an accessory for weekend or casual wear. Discreet skin and reptile surfaces can be worn for business, but it is safer to go for the timeless and durable, as well as top quality. College stripes, country motifs, rhinestones, and slogan belts are all fine for the appropriate occasion. Otherwise, as with shoes, over-designed and flashy belts are simply a recipe for style disaster.

Tip *Not being fashion items, quality leather accessories can be purchased whenever you find something suitable.*

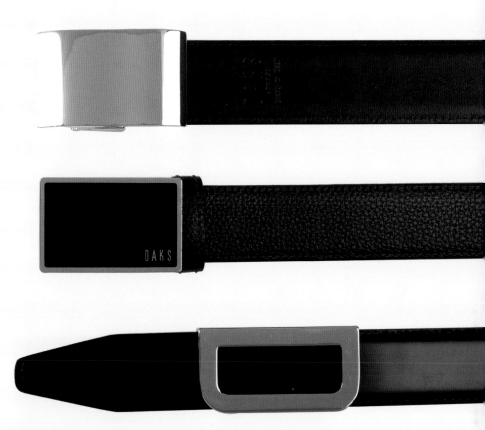

Above: Belts come in a wide range of styles. Having a selection allows you to change to suit the occasion.

SUSPENDERS Suspenders come in two styles: clip-on or button-on. If you wish to wear button-on suspenders, you will need to purchase trousers with the appropriate buttoning. The suspenders should always be of good quality webbing in a discreet color that goes with your suit, or for evening always in black. The ends forming either the support for the clip or the button extensions should be made of leather. Colored suspenders go in and out of fashion – but if you wish to wear them or find belts uncomfortable, the best advice is to stick to classic and understated.

TRAVEL DOCUMENTS Before traveling abroad, it is wise to invest in a good leather passport holder; this protects it from damage. Such a holder will often include a compartment for your boarding pass, saving a great deal of last-minute searching. A travel wallet that contains ticket, money, and passport is in theory a marvelous idea, but in practice if such a wallet is lost or stolen, you will have lost everything. It is advisable to have two or three containers: passport holder with boarding pass, wallet with tickets and schedules, and perhaps a third with hotel details and currency.

WATCHES

The advent of the cellular phone and the laptop computer, along with other personal technology items, has given a gentleman several options for checking the correct time. However, a wristwatch, or a selection of watches, can combine practicality with a style statement and also complete a top-to-toe look. Good classic watches may be costly, but over the years will not only provide pleasure for the wearer but, in time, be handed down to the next generation.

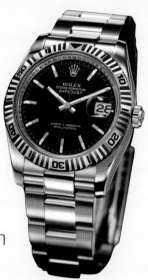

STATUS Status may derive from a famous watchmaker, a heritage style, or even a special handmade strap to wear the watch on. Whatever the case, make sure that you obtain value for your money with a versatile and adaptable style. One of the most sought-after watch designs available, the classic men's Rolex chronograph, is a heavy masculine watch with a metal strap. It needs little description, since a gentleman either desires one or doesn't.

Tip *Balance the size of your watch with your wrist size. If you have slim wrists, a huge heavy watch will look wrong, as will a small watch on a big wrist.*

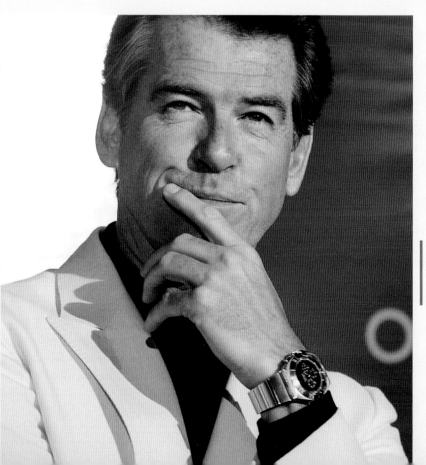

Left: *A watch is more than an accessory –it is a practical object as well as being a statement of status.*

SPORTS Any heavy-duty watch that is functional, shockproof, and waterproof will be suitable as a sports watch. Extra dials or specialized gauges will enhance the practicality for the wearer and possibly link it to a specific sporting activity. The strap may be either metal in a chunky style or sturdy webbing in nylon, perhaps with a sporty stripe motif. Different types of fastenings and dial shields can also be part of the sports watch.

TANK The classic oblong-faced watch, which, depending on the strap, may serve as both a business and a casual watch. Cartier created the "Tank" watch in 1917, inspired by the tanks from WW1. The iconic square or rectangular face, crossbar, and sidepieces, Roman numerals, and the faceted sapphire on the crown make the Cartier "Tank" watch instantly recognizable.

FUN DESIGNER These are watches with an easy relaxed style originally developed by the Swatch Company. Although some of the styles now look a little dated, the concept of the fun, colorful watch has remained and been developed in a variety of ways with decorative dials and straps.

DINNER/FORMAL For professional and red carpet occasions, a classic, understated style will complement a suit or tuxedo. Black leather watch straps suit both occasions and a neat classic dial with clear Roman numerals will make the correct style statement with formal clothing.

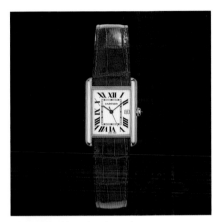
Above: City-chic, tank-style watch.

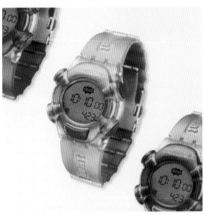
Above: Fun weekend and sports styles.

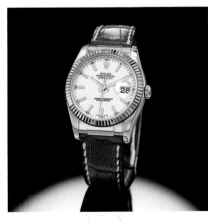
Above: Perfect style for the country.

GOLD OR STEEL If your coloring and appropriate color palette tend to the paler and cooler end of the spectrum, stick to steel; if warmer and stronger, go for gold.

LEATHER STRAPS An inexpensive watch can be upgraded by a top quality leather strap, but in all cases, the leather strap should be the best you can afford and changed whenever it looks tired and scruffy.

CARE Like anything mechanical, a watch requires care and servicing. The best option is to have at least two watches so that when one is being serviced you still have one to wear. Since watch styles follow fashion trends fairly slowly you can add to your collection and provide a rest for each watch. Having various watches suitable for a range of occasions will extend the life of each individual watch.

CELL PHONES, PERSONAL MUSIC SYSTEMS, AND ORGANIZERS In the modern life of a gentleman, other status symbols add to that of the watch. The gentleman should remember that these are personal items and should not annoy those around him: earphones should fit correctly into the ears; speaking loudly into cell phones or ostentatiously tapping at personal organizers and laptops are also signs of selfish behavior. A gentleman may have all the top-of-the-range technology at his fingertips, but it should be used discreetly, and cared for in a tidy manner.

JEWELRY & CUFF LINKS

Women may readily flaunt their accessories but a gentleman's opportunities for display of his jewelry are limited within modern style and culture.

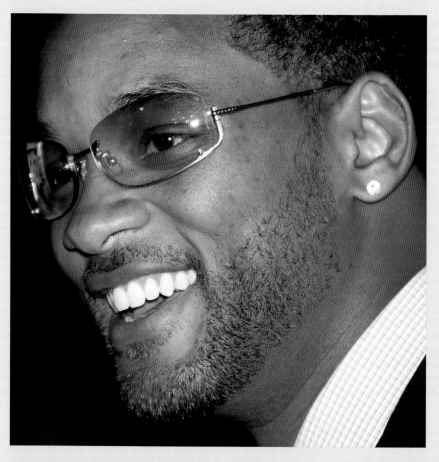

EARRINGS Throughout human history gentlemen have worn either a single earring or mismatched ear studs, although such ornaments are a little out of style at present. In general, a discreet gold circle through the ear or a small metal stud are the most acceptable. If you wish to wear either one or two earrings, make certain they may be worn during business hours.

Above: Ear studs are newer than ear rings and can be dazzling, as here, or something minimal and simple in gold.

Tip Always keep your cufflinks in their boxes ready to be worn or packed and not thrown in a heap in one container. When your links are all clumped together, not only will you be unable to locate pairs, but the links themselves may sustain damage.

NECKLACES For a man, the necklace may vary from a very fine gold chain to massive silver links. To match the chain, any ornaments attached should be in proportion to the links. The necklace can be precious and ancestral or simply stylish, but strictly for fun depending on the occasion and the style of the wearer. Many men regard the necklace as a nice way to hang on to souvenirs, such as a wedding ring, a tiny club shield in enamel, or a good luck symbol. Necklaces of shells, or thin leather laces with shell or decorative attachments, can be a great complement to a vacation outfit, and also show off a tan.

WRISTBANDS, CUFFS, & BRACELETS
From Ancient Greek warriors to the surfer dude of today, the wrist has been an area for adornment on many men. In the society of the twenty-first century, men can wear a fine gold chain next to a classic tank style watch during business hours or a bold ethnic bracelet with a sarong to the beach bar. Appropriateness is, as ever, the key to wrist jewelry. A heavy-link silver chain that looks great with a chunky sweater and jeans may look out of place at the office.

RINGS The signet or seal ring, especially when worn on the little finger, has a noble heritage since it is designed and created to enable a man to imprint his crest on sealing wax when closing a document. Times and habits may have changed, but for many men this is still one of the few items of jewelry they will countenance. A plain wedding band is also an acceptable style of ring for a man. The key indicator for the style and wearing of rings is suitability; a handful of heavy silver rings can look great, but not at the office with a formal suit. Gems are a great danger area in men's rings and can either look effeminate or flashy. If you are unsure, the best advice is to avoid them. If you wear any type of ring whatsoever, it will obviously draw attention to your hands, so be sure they deserve it by keeping them well manicured.

CUFF LINKS Aside from formal professional and red carpet cuff links, there are a great many design options, especially for casual wear. Motifs and references to sports, pursuits such as riding, and club symbols can make a classic, stylish yet individual statement for cuff links. Vintage and designer cuff links can enliven a dark weekend shirt, make a statement with jeans and a jacket for dinner, or demonstrate a special interest such as a sport or hobby. They may serve as a conversation piece as well as a functional cuff detail.

Tip If you are going to wear jewelry, keep it clean and repaired since, like everything you wear, it makes a statement about your sartorial style.

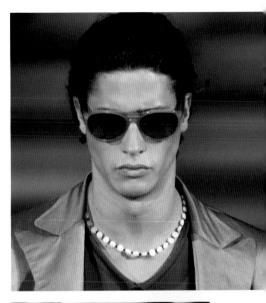

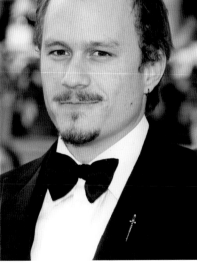

Above: *Summer is a great time for shell and bead neck bands. Keep them close to the neck and chunky in style for a masculine look (top). Jewels for men can often be classic in inspiration; this example is closer to a decoration or award than jewelry (above).*

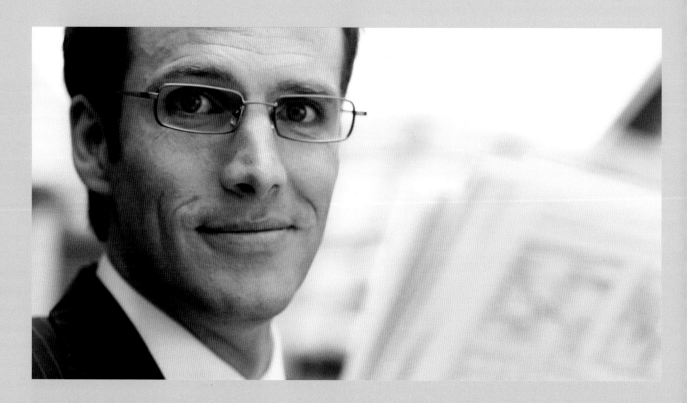

EYEWEAR

In spite of contact lenses, eye surgery, and major advances in ways to help people discard their glasses, eyewear remains an important daily fact of life to millions of men throughout the world. Since the earliest days of their invention, glasses have been subject to the whims of fashion. Since glasses are, by their positioning on the front of the face, such a style statement, it is essential to analyze your face shape before any other element can be decided upon. It is worth considering that an elaborate pair of statement designer spectacles will affect the impression you give to people both socially and professionally, so you need to consider this before making any decisions on what you buy.

FRAME SHAPE Look in the mirror to see that the outline of your face dictates the outline of your glasses frame. If you are unsure as to your face shape, draw around your reflection with some type of marker; the shape can then be analyzed. Round, oval, and square are the simple general shapes to work from, and once you know which one you have, you can select frames that harmonize with your face shape. If you have a round face, you do not want a round shape to exaggerate it; similarly, avoid a square frame on a square face. Trial and error with a range of styles in the final analysis is the way to search for a frame to suit you, along with the help of an informed and supportive salesperson.

Tip Sunglasses should be functional and flattering, so do not be tempted by fashion and a shape which does nothing to add to your overall style statement.

FEATURES A strong nose, small eyes, sharp cheekbones; whatever the strongest features are to your face they should be taken into account as the next step in your analysis of your face and the search for glasses that will enhance your appearance. Add this information to your face shape.

COLORING Finally, check your skin tone and hair color to enable you to select frames that complement your coloring. By adding these three elements together, you have knowledge of the background to your choice of glasses.

FRAMES You may visit as many optical stores as you wish, trying on and discussing frames with the staff until you find the store that has both the frames and staff you feel are right for you. Frames come in a dazzling array from big, bold, and black to clear and rimless, with every possible variation in between. Fashion also affects style and influences us to try new shapes, colors, and materials, although there will always be a few classic frame elements to consider.

TORTOISESHELL The mottled pattern frame materials are flattering and classic. In addition, they also come in a range of tones from very dark to pale, thus providing an option to suit most colorings, along with a variety of shapes and widths of frames. So you might buy a pair of spectacles in a dark tortoiseshell with a tiny round frame for an old-fashioned look, or a bold, blonde tortoiseshell in an oblong shape for a glamorous style.

PLAIN BLACK to colorless or transparent covers the range of plain colored frames to choose from, with almost every color of the rainbow in between. Obviously, flattering color is the first prerequisite in your selection and second is a classic, versatile shade to take you from suited formal through to casual weekend. In truth, although you may have several pairs of glasses, there will always be the newest or favorite pair that is worn most of the time.

SILVER, PEWTER, GOLD, GUNMETAL WIRE Whatever type of metallic color you can think of, someone makes frames in that shade. The clever thing is to choose a suitable metal in a suitable shape to work for you.

RIMLESS In theory, rimless frames should flatter everybody since they are created to disappear; this is far from the truth. Not only can the shape of the lens work for or against the face, but in many cases rimless glasses are aging since they offer neither color nor texture support to the face.

PARTIAL FRAMES This is a great alternative to fully rimless with just the upper part of the frame in metal, tortoiseshell, or plain color. The line created is bolder than rimless, but the rimless lower half lightens the effect. This style is both retro 50s and modern.

CASES If you do not wear your glasses all the time, you will require a case for them. Select one as carefully as any item in your wardrobe, and consider the occasions and functions you take your glasses to and purchase appropriate cases to complete your look. Leather for business, metal for weekends, and bright-colored nylon for vacation are just a few of the possibilities in design before you even start on pattern, texture, and the basic construction and style of the case. Glasses are another accessory that can make a surprisingly strong statement about your approach to style.

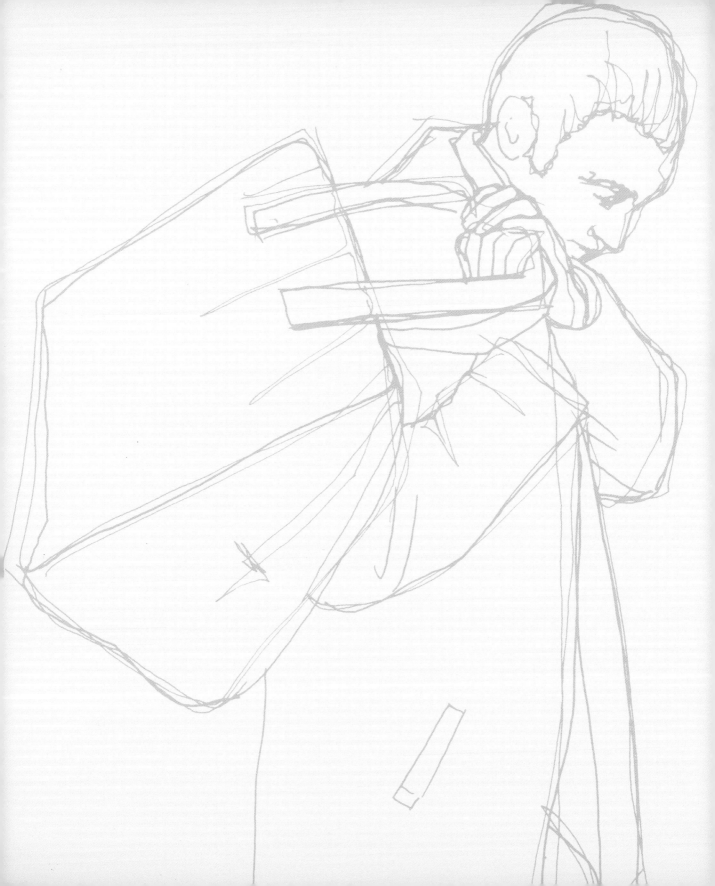

"In the Balkans they say that if you
long for faraway countries and leave
your own land and home to find them,
you are born under a lilac bleeding star."

LESLEY BLANCH, TRAVEL WRITER

BUSINESS TRAVEL

Just as life within your professional activities and at the workplace is made more pleasant and efficient through clarity, organization, and planning, so is the travel wardrobe. Throwing clothes into a suitcase until it is full, then jamming the lid shut or forcing the zipper around, will simply not do—it will only result in clothes that are both crumpled and uncoordinated. Simple organization and planning is all that is needed along with the application of a little common sense.

PLANNING The following elements should be written down as a guide for ease and effectiveness in your packing.

The first thing to do is note the length of the trip; the number of days and nights away; how many appointments and when and where they are; the number of times you might need to change or, more importantly, have the time and opportunity to change. There is no point in taking extra clothing that your schedule will not allow

you to wear. Starting with the facts is a key component in planning your packing. Now you know how many times you may change your clothes during the day, if at all, and second, you know the type of occasions for which you are packing. Next, work out simply what you need: start with the suits and remember that each suit will require a certain amount of room in your bag. If you are traveling in a business suit and going straight to a meeting, then decide which suit is most appropriate for both the journey and the meeting.

Write down how many shirts you will need, allowing a spare for accidents, and the same with socks, underwear, ties, and so on. If you have a hectic schedule, nothing restores your equilibrium like a few minutes for a quick shower, perhaps a second shave, and to follow, fresh clothes from top to toe.

Left: To arrive looking good when traveling for business requires wardrobe planning, careful packing and appropriate luggage and bags.

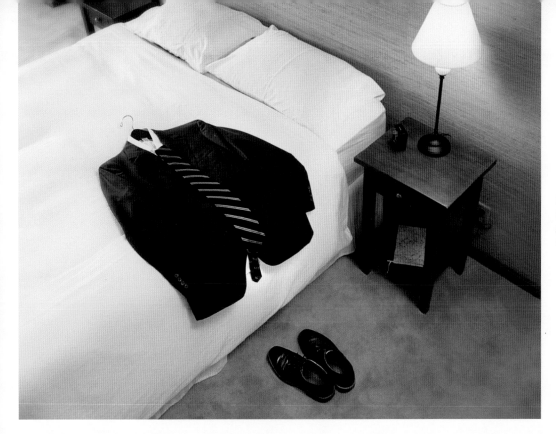

Left: *If you prepare your travel wardrobe carefully, getting dressed is fast, efficient, and easy.*

PACKING When you have worked out the fewest items you can take, lay everything out to gauge the packing required. Options in luggage are essential to provide suitable flexibility with your packing. A suit carrier, a hard-top suitcase on wheels, a large zippered carry-all, a small carry-on bag: whatever your choices, make sure they are clean and properly labeled. Investing in good luggage tags can help identify your baggage and make it look more businesslike. Bear in mind that suit bags are useful items of luggage, but will not hold everything and if too full will actually crease your clothes.

Toiletries should be transferred to small lightweight bottles and, if possible, placed in your carry-on bag with socks and underwear wrapped around them. Shoes are the heaviest item to pack for a trip, so they must be kept to the minimum number of pairs. Based on the shoe appropriate for the main suit of the trip, wear one pair, perhaps a slip-on style for travel, and pack a lace-up pair. Remember to take a shoe-cleaning kit with you; it weighs nothing and takes up very little space, yet if you are wearing the same pair of shoes fairly often, it keeps them looking fresh and clean.

Tip If you travel a great deal, keep a spare toiletry bag ready and filled to save time when packing.

HOW TO PACK When packing, plastic is as effective as tissue paper, so place dry-cleaning bags between layers of clothes to trap the air between them and help prevent creasing. Fold and layer your clothes neatly when packing or, as an alternative, roll your clothes for packing ready to be unrolled on arrival, perhaps even leaving wire coat hangers in the garments. Fold each garment as few times as possible to maximize space in the suitcase. Jackets should be buttoned up, the sleeves straight down the main body of the garment and the entire jacket simply folded in half. Trousers and shirts should also be folded in half; with shirts, fold the sleeves straight across the chest. Once they are folded, garments can be stacked by weight to avoid crushing, with jackets first at the bottom, then trousers, and finally the shirts and other lightweight items on top. Fill out the corners of the suitcase with rolled ties, cufflink boxes, socks, and underwear.

Tip If unsure about evening events, pack a dark suit, dressy white shirt, and a bow tie.

BUSINESS TRAVEL

Having planned your days, the events, and the type of clothing you need to pack, it is important to ascertain if the clothes selected will get you through without unnecessary weight.

FORMAL PLANNING Planning a formal business trip is simple and straightforward and should be done stage by stage. First, hang up the suit or jacket and trousers you plan to travel in. Next add the shirt, sweater, and coat, even the scarf and shoes, if appropriate. This is your starting point and may be changed as you plan. Next, put beside this outfit the suit you plan to wear for business and add the shirt, tie, and so on, then repeat until you have laid out all the clothes you judge necessary, at this stage, to cover the trip. Now analyze what you have selected and start to edit or exchange so that there is less than you started with. Even if there are three different events during a day, there is no need for three suits, three shirts, and three ties. Other lightweight and easy-to-pack accessories such as scarves, cufflinks, or even a vest will change the appearance of a classic suit. Figure out how two suits can be exchanged and re-accessorized to work in different ways so as to last over three days.

Right: Good packing is an art, but if you are a frequent business traveler it is an art which it pays to learn. With time, care, and consideration it is amazing what one item of luggage can contain.

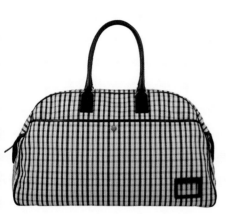

Above: Bold check helps this bag to stand out and the easy-grip handles and neat identification tag are strictly practical.

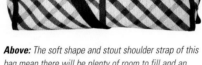

Above: The soft shape and stout shoulder strap of this bag mean there will be plenty of room to fill and an comfortable way of carrying it.

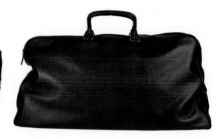

Above: Luxury styling and fabric combined with a neat shape mean this bag is most appropriate for shorter business trips.

LUGGAGE & BAGGAGE As mentioned before, it is important to have a selection of bags and suitcases to accommodate varying lengths of trip and amounts to be packed. This includes travel bags, briefcases, and other bags, such as the case for your laptop computer. There is no sadder sight than a well-dressed business man at the airport or train station encumbered with a suit bag, a carry-all, a briefcase, and a computer bag; what is even sadder is that there is no need for this assortment of baggage if forethought is applied while packing. In this case, a large soft zippered bag could contain the suits and the rest of the clothing, with an external zippered compartment capable of holding the briefcase, and one carry-all containing the computer inside in a padded wallet. If the idea is to avoid checking your baggage, or to cram everything into a small space, the dexterity and loss of temper required to cope with the multi-bag option seems poor planning indeed. Huge computer bags and oversized briefcases should be purged before a business trip, when only the essentials should be carried. Ascertain what equipment will be at the offices you are visiting. Technology means we should be able to take a presentation on a disk, e-mail papers ahead for copying, check on requirements, and so on, rather than assuming our own equipment is unique and indispensable.

Tip Since they are not fashion items, always buy classic quality luggage and baggage in preparation for future travel.

TOILETRIES It is good to know that in this day and age you can buy toothpaste almost anywhere in the world. This means that if you forget something, it is not the end of the world. The requirements for a toiletry bag are shaving gel, razor, after-shave balm, toothbrush, toothpaste, shampoo, hair treatment, deodorant, and fragrance. Include cotton swabs, lip balm, and any special treatment applications to a total of thirteen items at most. If all of these are placed into plastic travel-size bottles, it should not be necessary to use a huge bag to contain them. A good stout toiletry bag, especially if you travel regularly on business, is a wise investment since it will protect both the contents and the clothes with which it may be packed. Do not act under the illusion that a plastic bag filled with an assortment of bottles and cans will never let you down; it is false economy.

Tip If you can, buy travel sizes of your regular toiletries when you see them and keep them ready for use in the future.

VACATION TRAVEL

Many of the rules for business travel apply equally to vacation travel; in fact, it is even more important to plan your time ahead and to select the appropriate wardrobe for your trip.

WHAT TYPE OF VACATION? There are many varieties of vacation, from a glamorous capital weekend on the other side of the world to a long, lazy summer holiday on the coast. There are sightseeing vacations and active sporting trips. Summer and winter trips and vacations can vary in length from Friday to Sunday to a month of travel. Each trip requires its own planning and the accompanying wardrobe can help make it a success or an endless vista of vacation sartorial disasters. So decide, once you have booked and arranged your vacation, what sort of wardrobe will meet all the requirements of the occasions likely to occur during your time away.

Tip Pack as carefully for a vacation as you would for a business trip and you will be rewarded with a trouble-free wardrobe. Throw it all in at the last minute and you will be rewarded with a bag of the wrong clothes and the need to go shopping when you arrive.

Right: *Vacation can mean town and more formal locations as well as beach and sea. Sharp pieces in crisp fabrics, yet worn and styled in a relaxed way, are perfect in this situation.*

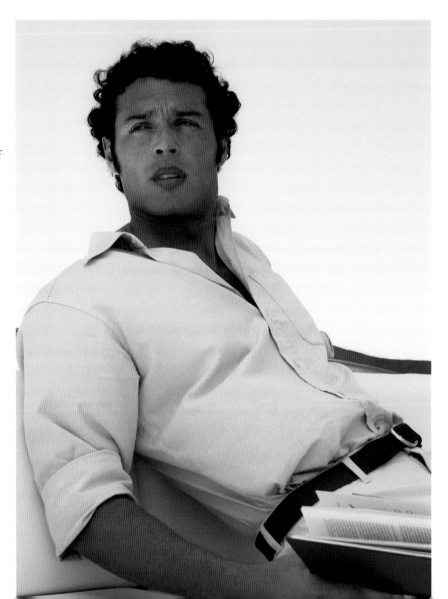

CITY VERSUS BEACH Lazy days on the beach or by the pool require little more than swimwear, some shirts and shorts and, if you have the style, some sarongs. (Note: While sarongs may be anathema to some men, they are practical, comfortable wear, and can be thrown down on to the sand instead of a towel. So before you decline the offer of a sarong, think about it.) Shoes can be the basic thong sandal or flip-flop, consisting of a sole and two straps, which are really only worn to stop your feet from getting burned or chafed. Evenings in town, at a restaurant, bar, or club require trousers, shirts, and footwear a step up from the beach shoe. Jackets may not be needed, but if you do require one, make sure it is suitable, in an unstructured style closer to a shirt than a suit jacket. Stick to just one or two colors for your vacation wardrobe and everything will mix and match over the days. A wardrobe based on green and sand might work in the following way: a long pair of khaki cotton shorts, khaki military-style cotton trousers, and two pairs of linen drawstring trousers: one dark green, the other pale sand. Add a mid-tone greenish sand linen jacket and some khaki, green, and sand undershirts and T-shirts. Complete the look with a dark green jungle print sarong and some sand and khaki shirts with long sleeves, which can be rolled up as necessary. Then add beach shoes and lightweight casual shoes along with sneakers or boots for travel and sightseeing. Finally, don't forget swimwear, underwear, and toiletry bag. Add multiples of any of these items and you are still well prepared for a vacation of varying occasions. Accessories such as belts and hats will add to your outfits (and, of course, you may purchase some extras while away).

> *Tip* *Make sure that any town visits do not include the need for a more formal outfit for evenings. A smart shirt and tie tucked in your suitcase may help out in such an eventuality.*

CITY VACATIONS *See City Casual.*
COUNTRY *See Country Dressing.*
SPORTING TRIPS *See Sportswear.*

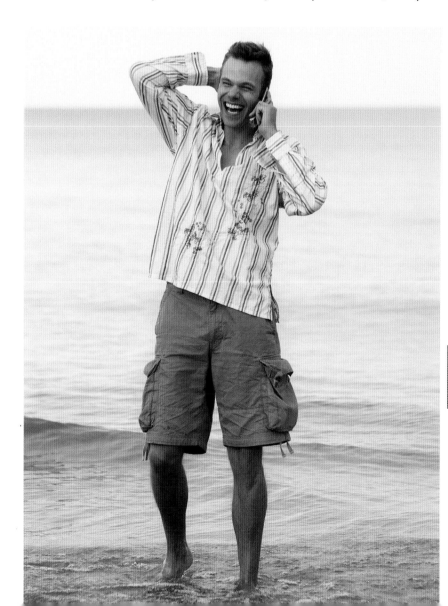

Left: *East fit, but not baggy or oversized, the cool colors and simple pieces of this outfit would look at easy at the bar, on the beach, or sightseeing.*

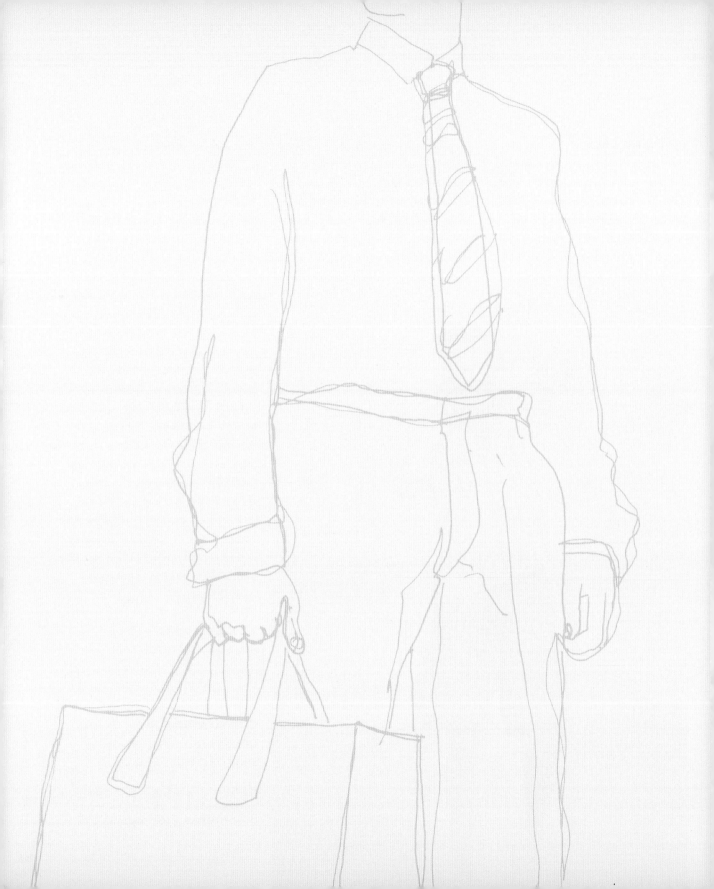

"Instead of a collection of jackets and trousers, which you would have in a range, in a collection all the individual parts go together and something ties them, whether it is color or texture or silhouette."

PAUL SMITH, FASHION DESIGNER

PUTTING IT ALL TOGETHER

COORDINATION

Although it would seem that any fool with a wardrobe of the right clothes could get dressed in the morning and leave home looking good, life is, rather unfairly, not that simple. Combining garments, accessories, and the occasion requires consideration, application, and organization, and this where some rules are helpful and supportive.

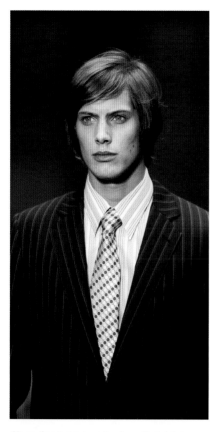

Above: Smart, classic, and well coordinated, but without a hint of being dull, boring, and conventional. It is all in the planning of the outfit.

Appropriate dress, along with the accompanying grooming, is vital to make a gentleman feel confident and comfortable.

Getting dressed to go to work might include an overcoat, suit, shirt, tie, cufflinks, belt, shoes, socks, and briefcase. Each and every component of this outfit must be considered and should be in harmony with all the other elements; a tall order indeed.

FORMAL COLOR Be careful of too much color matching. Blue on blue on blue will add up shade by shade to become stronger in total color. Contrast of tones will help, but even the smallest accent of color will break up the over-coordinated look of the outfit. If the blue is very dark, black shoes and briefcase and a dark tie with a navy and black pattern are appropriate. If it is a lighter navy suit, it may be accented with lilac, rose pink, or soft lemon. Dark brown may be lifted with a fine touch of orange or dark leaf green,

perhaps in a tie or cufflinks. Often a fine stripe, fleck, or check, in either the suit fabric or shirt, will suggest an accent shade.

FORMAL FABRIC Texture and surface can impart a level of freshness as well as style panache. The matte quality of a suit fabric, with a soft cotton shirt and the added richness and sheen of a silk tie, is fairly classic; but perhaps shine and sheen can be added in other ways. The cotton shirt might have a subtle satin stripe, or perhaps the tie has matte and shine in the fabric structure. The metal of cufflinks and even the shine of polished leather for shoes and briefcase all add contrast to a complete look. It is the addition of every element to the next that creates the impact, not each item in isolation.

Tip When layering clothes, you may find that your size varies. Your T-shirt may be medium and your sweatshirt large or a sweater in medium fits well over a small T-shirt.

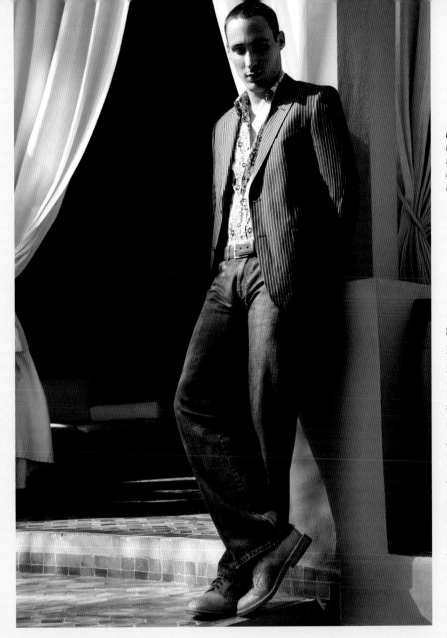

Left: *This gentleman looks relaxed and stylish with a hint of the dandy, but still understated and classic. In fact this look would be at home in town or country, for informal business or on vacation; by breaking some rules it makes a versatile style statement.*

SILHOUETTE In combinations, the rule is simple: when adding layers from the first item closest to the body, the size should increase to the outer layers. Although this seems obvious in practice, remember not to wear a baggy undershirt under a slim-cut sweatshirt or a slim-cut vest over a baggy shirt. The result is both untidy and enlarging when bulky fabric is trapped in lumps under a slimmer outer layer. The body pieces such as T-shirts and undershirts, and even shirts and sweats, should be worn with the next garment lying smoothly over them rather than suppressing them. Stuffing the baggy sleeves of a heavy knit sweater into a too-tight jacket or coat can only result in discomfort. This seemingly obvious advice is about both the visual unattractiveness and the physical awkwardness that will result if you ignore it.

Tip When shopping, check out the new stores; don't just stick to your old favorites. You may or may not purchase anything, but it will refresh your view of the stores you do frequent and give you an idea of other available styles.

CITY CASUAL LOOKS

The impact of fabric and color combinations in putting outfits together may be fully explored in casual urban attire. The spring example could be a shirt in cool blue cotton, a dark navy V-neck sweater, a navy pinstriped suit jacket, and dark indigo jeans. Add a purple and lilac-striped cotton knit scarf and black polished boots with a blue and gray nylon messenger bag. The Autumn version could be a pale lilac shirt, a dark purple V-neck sweater, a rich brown corduroy coat, and dark indigo jeans. The additions would be a purple, brown, and lilac mohair scarf, dark brown boots, and a textured brown leather messenger bag. In both examples note how texture and color combine and how colors used twice in differing shades hold the outfit together.

COORDINATION

COUNTRY LOOKS

There is an easy and simple rule to remember for dressing for the country: don't pretend to be someone you are not. Put simply, if you wear full riding gear people will assume you ride, and if you don't ride but dress as if you do, then you will certainly look a fool. Cowboy, farmhand, fisherman, and landowner are all legitimate occupations out of town, but unless they are your real reasons for being in the country, please avoid role play within your wardrobe. For most people visiting the country a classic, functional wardrobe will serve its purpose.

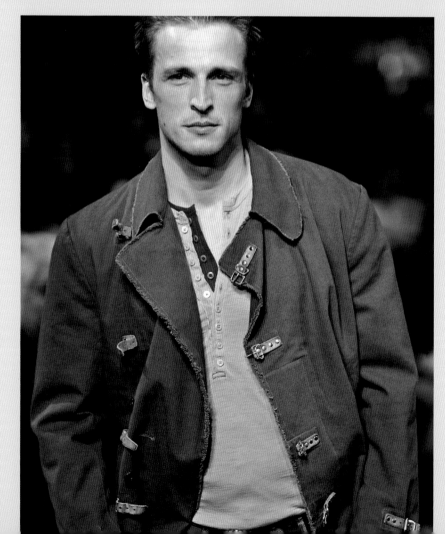

DAY-TO-DAY, OUT AND ABOUT

Comfortable trousers, a jacket with weatherproof properties, and an easy shirt will provide the basics for any country outfit. This might mean brushed cotton, corduroy, tweed, or military-inspired trousers; a tweed, corduroy, or waxed cotton jacket; and a shirt in heavy cotton or even fine-needle corduroy. Worn with either a stout shoe or a short boot, the style of these combinations is casual but not specific to a particular occupation. Depending on the season, sweaters, scarves, gloves and even a coat as an added layer will provide a basic country wardrobe.

Left: *Easy and practical country pieces based on good quality fabrics and colors make a style statement.*

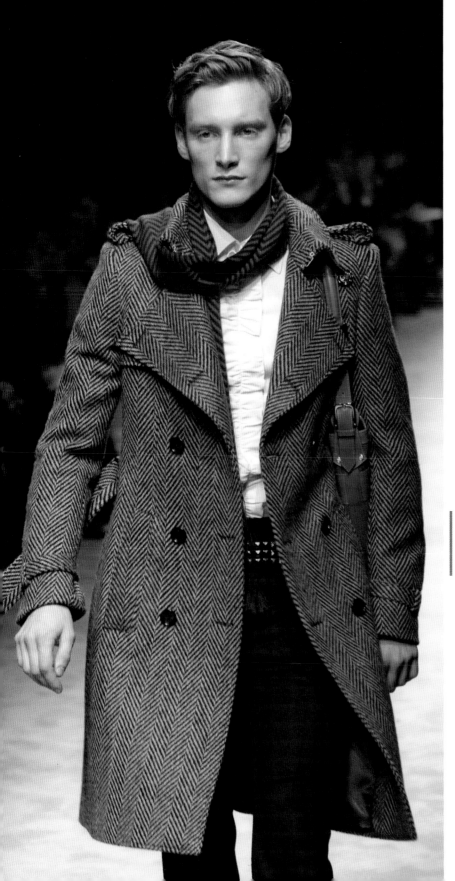

Left: Country dandy combines with creative dressing in classic items using strong fabrics and colors. Individually each piece is relatively low-key; it is the combination which makes this a stand-out look.

COUNTRY TOWN Visiting a country town in any season may involve shopping, lunch, or perhaps a visit to a sporting club. The jacket is often the key to looking a touch more formal than when out in the countryside. Try to have a shirt which is a bit crisper in fabric and styling and which, when combined with khakis, jeans, or corduroy trousers, means the top half of the outfit is semi-formal. The signal you wish to send out is relaxed and easy, but still based on formal components, thus making a subtle statement of regard for the fact it is town, but in the country, and you understand the requirements of dress appropriate to this milieu.

Tip When spending a weekend in the country, do check out the evening activities. Some country establishments can be a bit grand, so it is best to be prepared.

COUNTRY EVENING Clothing for the evening in the country can on occasion be pretty dressy, but as a general rule this is a time when you might wish to be a touch more creative with color and fabric. Perhaps select a rich or dark-colored velvet or corduroy for either the jacket or trousers and team them with something plain. The addition of a colored shirt with a plain jacket can be perfect for dinner. The total effect is formal but relaxed and just a touch down from dressing for dinner in town.

CREATIVE DRESSING AND COLOR

It is fair to assume that if you are an extrovert and center-stage type of dresser, you would not be reading the advice within these pages. However, some of you may wish to be a little more "classic with a twist" in style, or simply prefer a more designer-led wardrobe, but are unsure how to go about it or what guidelines to follow.

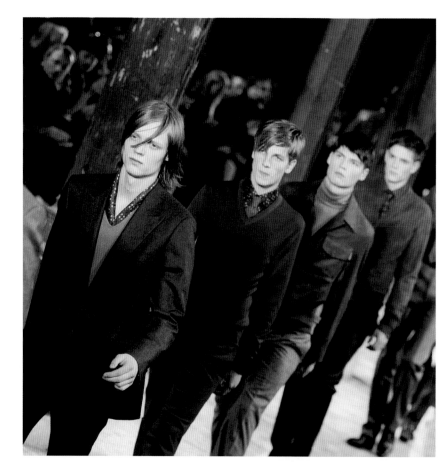

BALANCE The key to successful creative dressing is never to over-style from top to toe with every element fighting for attention. Each creative piece should be carefully teamed with something quiet and classic to complement and offset it.

Interesting details on a jacket should not be backed up by a quirky shirt, an artistic tie, and detailed trousers. The detailed jacket will work much better with a classic shirt, neat coordinated tie, and some simple trousers, all selected in fabrics that harmonize.

The bold silhouette of a suit will make a strong enough statement as it stands, without resorting to "gilding the lily" by adding a loud patterned tie and wildly colored shirt.

Left: Use bright colors as accents, as you would flavors in cooking—spiced but not overseasoned.

COLOR & FABRIC Simple additions are often key to putting creative looks together, and color and fabric can be especially successful here. Perhaps an unexpected color combination for suit and shirt, such as a rich dark brown and dark violet, or dark navy and shell pink, or pale silver gray and ice blue. Perhaps when selecting suit fabrics for custom tailoring, you will find a fabric with a bold color within the weave that could be made into a classic suit, or a classic fabric to have made or to purchase in a new silhouette. Linings in bold colors have already been mentioned, but teaming the lining with a matching or complementary tie or scarf is a subtle way of creative color that is only emphasized when the jacket lining is revealed.

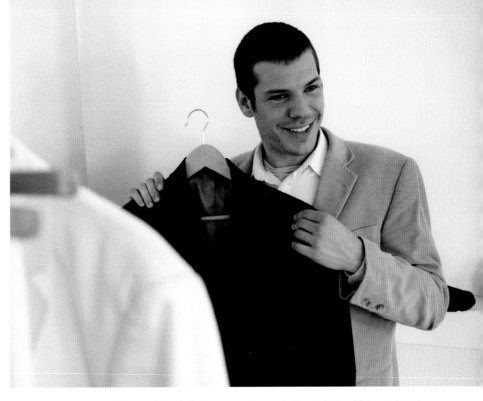

Above: The color spectrum offers a confusing choice, but once you have worked out the basics of light or dark, cool or warm and so on, you can then experiment with creative, flattering shades and combinations.

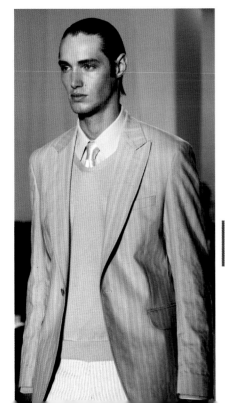

PLANNING As always, try laying clothes out to see the effect. This can lead to making more interesting combinations from a fairly classic wardrobe, as well as generating ideas for extra purchases that will make your style a little more creative. A new color for suits, a rich woven scarf, or a change of color for a formal shirt can add just the creative touch to your style that will demonstrate thought and an eye for detail, rather than screaming out "Fashion victim!"

Tip A fabric that incorporates several shades of the same color can be more versatile than a fabric with too many different colors.

Left: Soft and pale colors can actually be bold in their impact and the statement they make visually.

Check style publications for tips on the newest pieces to add color. If you have friends who are more creative dressers than you (successful ones, that is) try some of their clothes to get fresh ideas. This is part of the process of planning creative dressing top to toe—experiment. Spend some time in stores that stock new creative designers. Observe what the other customers try, and experiment with new elements for your wardrobe. You are under no obligation to buy—keep shopping until you are 100 percent sure that the color, detail, silhouette, or fabric is just what you need for your wardrobe—then, and only then, purchase. Remember, if you make a mistake, if you hate it when you get it home, if it doesn't work as you thought it would, take it back. It is a complete waste of money to let it hang unworn in your closet.

GLOSSARY

anorak Hip-length. Inuit-inspired hooded jacket.

blazer Double-breasted with metal buttons is the key style, but since its creation at the beginning of the 20th century, the blazer has been striped, single-breasted, and otherwise modified as fashion and style dictate.

bomber jacket The bomber jacket, golf jacket, and windbreaker are all short jackets with a zippered front and a high enclosed neck for warmth and protection. They usually have two pockets and are lined for warmth. May have a ribbed trim.

brocade Fabric with a weave that creates a raised pattern.

brogue The holes punched into the decoration on a classic leather shoe are characteristic of the brogue.

brushed cotton Soft cotton fabric with a brushed surface. May come in heavyweight cottons.

button-down The collar of this shirt has two buttonholes to fasten to corresponding buttons sewn to the body of the shirt.

caftan An ancient garment that is today a cut-over shirt in tunic style that pulls on over the head. Popular for resort and vacation wear, it may be short and colorful in crisp cotton or long and floating in basic black or white.

cardigan Named after the Earl of Cardigan (1797–1868), this is a knitted jacket that fastens down the front. Varies in its fashionability like many classic garments and is transformed by changes in silhouette.

Chesterfield Named in the 1830s after Lord Chesterfield, this was originally a gray fitted coat with black velvet collar; today it is seen in a variety of styles.

covert coat Covert is a soft but firmly woven wool fabric; this coat generally comes in rustic shades from pale camel to deep green.

cummerbund Worn in the 19th century as a substitute for the waistcoat, or vest, this was originally a waist sash but today is closer to a deep belt in style.

double-face A cloth created with two sides that may be two different colors or two different types, such as shiny on one side and matte on the other.

drainpipe trousers Narrow, close-to-the-leg trousers that often wrinkle around the knee and ankle.

duffle coat Short coat, generally with a hood, originally worn during WWII and characterized by the toggle fastening and heavy woolen fabric.

evening pumps (or dancing shoes) A Victorian shoe, still worn for formal occasions. Available both in highly polished and patent leather, it has a rounded to square toe, small heel, and a scoop front decorated with a flat bow.

flannel A tightly woven wool fabric with a slightly brushed surface.

gabardine Fine twill surfaced fabric.

gingham A classic check of alternating squares in white and color; often found in shirts.

Harris tweed Tweed woven on the isle of Harris, Scotland.

Hawaiian Traditional prints and motifs that decorate shirts and shorts. The bold colors and often amusing motifs lead many men to overindulge this look, which is unkind to the larger stomach and overpowering on a small physique.

herringbone Pattern of diagonal and reversed diagonal lines creating arrow-shaped patterning.

hipster Hipster trousers (or hiphuggers) ride on the hip bone with a short rise to them.

intarsia A technique to place motifs and patterns in knitwear.

jacquard A technique for machine-made patterns in knitwear.

jodhpurs Riding breeches named after a city in India.

kilt Identified with Scotland since the 17th century, this garment has become a classic. Either in a clan tartan or plain wool, the kilt can be worn to any number of formal occasions as a style statement.

lapel Front of the jacket which turns back to form the collar.

Levis After some years of producing variations, Levi Strauss patented jeans in 1872 and added copper rivets in 1873.

linen Woven from natural plant fibers, this fabric is characterized by easy creasing of the surface and suitability for warm climates.

loden Traditional dark green Tyrolean fabric from Austria used for making coats.

Lycra Patented elastic yarn used for added stretch in clothing.

madras Brightly checked fabric from India.

mohair Fiber from the Angora goat, popular in the 1950s for sharp suit material with a shine to the surface.

Nehru jacket Named after Pandit Nehru (1889–1964), this slim jacket fastening to a stand collar has become almost a classic for men who prefer not to wear evening shirts and bow ties.

Norfolk jacket The Norfolk jacket named after the Duke of Norfolk is a style with an integral belt and pleats. Late 19th century style, which is revived from time to time; is difficult to wear with confidence.

parka Longer, looser version of the anorak.

patch pocket The pocket is laid onto the body of the garment and attached by stitching.

plus fours Trousers or knickerbockers fastened just below the knee, popular in the 1920s. Verging on costume attire, they are difficult to wear with confidence in contemporary society.

polo shirt Traditionally a short-sleeved knitted shirt worn for sports, this style now comes in long-sleeve, jersey, and even sweatshirt variations.

polyester Synthetic fiber that creates crease-resistant and drip-dry fabric.

raglan Named after Lord Raglan (1788–1855), the sleeves on this garment are cut with part of the body to allow greater freedom of movement.

reefer jacket (or pea jacket) Generally double-breasted nautical-style jacket in navy with either matching or metal buttons. Originally worn by sailors in the 19th century.

revers The lapel on a coat or jacket.

rise The length of the seam running under the crotch is measured by the length from chair to waist when seated. The cut of trousers can be uncomfortable if the rise does not fit.

seersucker Cotton fabric with puckered stripes running through it, popular for summer jackets and blazers.

self color Any addition in the same color as the main fabric.

self pattern Motifs or patterns in the same color as the main fabric.

shawl collar A smooth curved collar with no indentations.

silk Luxury yarn produced from the cocoons of silk worms.

smoking jacket A Victorian jacket in an elaborate fabric, often belted, designed to be worn at home.

suede The skin side of a hide brushed to form a velvety surface.

tanga A tiny brief with string sides and sometimes no back, similar to a posing pouch as worn by nude models for modesty.

tartan Scottish check in tough woolen cloth created to identify each separate clan.

tone on tone Where the pattern is in a similar shade to the base color.

trenchcoat Military-style coat based on 19th century style with shoulder-loops and a double yoke. Generally in gabardine or lightweight wool.

tuxedo Named after The Tuxedo Club in New Jersey, this jacket can be single- or double-breasted with silk lapels.

twill Fabric woven with diagonal lines or ridges.

vent The single or double split at the back of a jacket. Originally for ease on horseback and to allow room for the sword.

vest A sleeveless jacket worn as a layer; also known as a waistcoat. The classic style has small buttons down the front, two pockets, and a half belt to adjust for fit at the back. Traditionally the bottom button is left unfastened for chic.

vintage Secondhand, antique, or recycled clothing is now generally known as vintage, meaning it had a previous life before the current wearer purchased it.

viscose A man-made fiber derived from wood pulp. Often used for T-shirts, summer shirts, and scarves.

waistcoat See vest.

yoke The panel of fabric across the shoulders of a garment, which may be front, back, or both. Shirt yokes at the back allow movement without bulk.

FURTHER READING

85 Ways to Tie a Tie: The Science and Aesthetics of Tie Knots
Thomas Fink
(HarperCollins Publishers, 2001)

The Allure of Men
Francois Baudot
(Assouline, 2000)

Brioni (Universe of Fashion)
Farid Chenoune
(Universe, 1998)

Cuff Links
Susan Jonas
(Harry N Abrams, 1991)

Elements of Style
Phillip Bloch
(Warner Books, 1998)

Handmade Shoes for Men
Lasz Vass
Konemann, 2002

Henry Poole: Founders of Savile Row: The Making of a Legend
Stephen Howarth
(Bene Factum Publishers, 2003)

The Indispensable Guide to Classic Men's Clothing
Christopher Sulavik
(Tatra Press, 1999)

Men of Color: Fashion, History, Fundamentals
Quincy Jones
(Artisan, 1998)

Mistakes Men Make That Women Hate: 101 Style Tips for Men
Kenneth J. Karpinski
(Capital Books, 2003)

The Modern Gentleman: A Guide to Essential Manners, Savvy & Vice
Phineas Mollod, Jason Tesauro
(Ten Speed Press, 2002)

Off the Cuff: The Guy's Guide to Looking Good
Carson Kressley
(Plume, 2005)

Style and the Man: How and Where to Buy the Best Men's Clothes
Alan Flusser
(HarperCollins, 1996)

The Suit: A Machiavellian Approach to Men's Style
Nicholas Antongiavanni
(Collins, 2006)

A Well-Dressed Gentleman's Pocket Guide
Oscar Lenius
(Trafalgar Square Publishing, 1998)

INDEX

ACKNOWLEDGMENTS

AUTHOR ACKNOWLEDGMENTS

To my father, Leslie, who provided a sartorial template, to my mother, Joan, who encouraged me to buy the hundreds of books that supported the writing of this book, and to Thomass Atkinson and Sheelagh Wright for their patience. To Geraldine Clark, Josie Wye, Lorna Selby, David Downton, Paul Ziolkowski, and Mark Andrew James for their support and advice.

PICTURE ACKNOWLEDGMENTS

The publisher would like to thank Gresham Blake (www.greshamblake.com) for the kind loan of props for photography. The publisher would also like to thank the following organizations for the use of images in this book. Every effort has been made to acknowledge the pictures, however we apologize if there are any unintentional omissions.

American Crew: 12 left

Aqua di Parma: 17

Aquascutum: 58

Aramis Lab Series: 10

Austin Reed: 63 bottom

Cartier Ltd: 151 top

Comfort Zone, www.comfortzone.it: 15

Corbis: Leland Bobbe: 11 bottom; Brooke Fasani: 11 top right; Jose Louis Pelaez, Inc: 18 top; Jim Cornfield: 19 right; Randy Faris: 21; P. Winbladh/zefa: 24 right; Miles/zefa: 25; Holger Scheibe/zefa: 26, 35 bottom right; Creasource: 27 top; Cynthia Hart Designer: 28 bottom; Barry Seidman: 28 top; Uwe Krejci/zefa: 34 bottom right; Shift Photo/zefa: 35 top left; Brian Bailey: 36; Serge Kroughlikoff/zefa: 37 top; Condé Nast Archive: 48 middle; Rolf Bruderer: 52; Annabel Williams: 54; Newmann/zefa: 57; Anthony Redpath: 58; Lawrence Manning: 59; Ansgar/zefa: 62, 171 top; Grace/zefa: 63 top, 137 left; stock4B: 82, 117 left; Hirdes/zefa: 84; H.G. Rossi/zefa: 86; C. Lyttle/zefa: 108; Dale C. Spartas: 109 right; Mitchell Layton/NewSport: 114; Michael Prince: 130; SIE Productions/zefa: 141, 138-9; Javier Pierini: 146; Bettmann: 147; Devan/zefa: 154; LWA-sharie Kennedy/zefa: 163; Emmanuel Fradin/Reuters: 171 bottom

DAKS: 42, 48 top, 49, 83, 89 left, 89 right, 93 left, 101, 127, 136, 148, 149, 161, back cover

Frangi Tie Rack: 82

Getty Images: Francesco Bittichesu: 1; Serge Krouglikoff: 6; Jonathan Knowles: 7; Don Klumpp: 11 left; Taxi: 14, 23, 88; Adie Bush: 17 middle; Mark Lewis: 30; Christopher Bissell: 32; Steve Smith: 35 top right; Brooke Fasani/Photonica: 37 bottom; Getty Images: 48 bottom, 87, 93 bottom right, 106, 116, 132, 151 middle; Altrendo: 51, 63 top centre, 106; Ray Kachatorian: 56; AFP: 63 bottom centre, 133, 150, 166, 168, 169, 170; Fernanda Calfat: 92 left, 94 right, 107; Kristian Dowling: 92 right, 109 middle; Thos Robinson: 94 left; Giuseppe Cacace: 95, 97, 124, 125, 131, 153 top right; Photonica: 96; Homer Sykes: 100; Alexander Walter: 105 bottom; Gary Hubbell: 109 left; Tom Stock: 111 left; Ronald Martinez: 115 top; Arthur Tilley: 115 left; Bernhard Lang: 117 right; Fredrik Clement: 118; Hassan Kinley: 119; Markus Boesch: 120; Harry Sheridan: 121; Time Life Pictures: 128; Harald Eisenberger: 129; Kelvin Murray: 137 right; Tseisuke Shinoda: 148; Frederick M. Brown: 152; Frazer Harrison: 153 bottom right; John Lund: 159; J. Christopher Lawson: 160; Bruce Laurance: 162

Guerlain: 17, 33 left

Henry Poole & Co, Savile Row: 75

Jaeger, 01553 732102: 85 bottom, 111 right, 167

Jones Bootmaker, 0800 163519: 50 bottom, 85 middle

JupiterImages Corporation: 27 bottom, 55

Kobal Collection/Danjaq/eon/UA: 33 right; Engstead: 53

Loake Shoemakers, www.loake.co.uk: 50 top, 85 top, 110, 142

The North Face: 89 middle

Pringle of Scotland Collection: 102, 103, 105 top

Remmington: 18 bottom left, 19 left, 20 left, right, 21 inset, 34 bottom left, top left, top right

Rex Features/Sunset: 78; Nils Jorgensen: 80; Snap: 143

RichardAndersonLtd.com: 43, 46, 64, 66, 74 left, 74 right, 76, 138 left

Rolex UK, www.Rolex.com: 150 top left, 151 bottom

Smythson: 58 inset

Geo. F. Trumper, London, www.trumpers.com: 12, 13, 16, 17, 22 left, right, 26 inset, 31 bottom

Lena White, www.lenawhite.co.uk: 29, 31 top